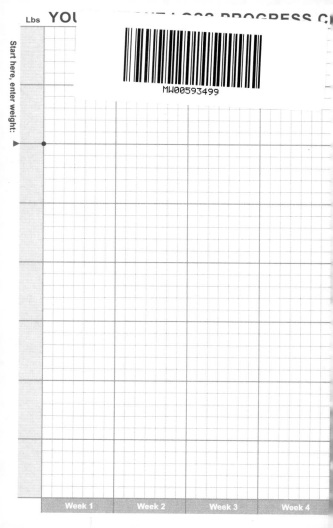

program as you gradually achieve your weight-loss goals.

HART

Chart your daily and/or weekly progress over the course of y

Week 5   Week 6   Week 7   Week 8

gram as you gradually achieve your weight-loss goals.

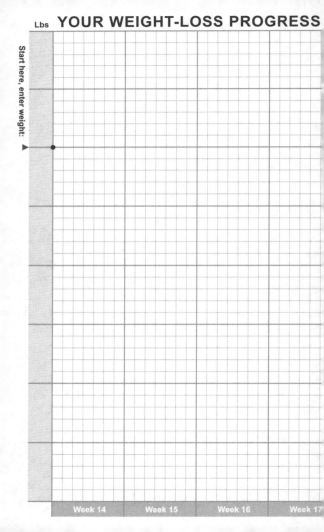

YOUR WEIGHT-LOSS PROGRESS

Lbs

Start here, enter weight:

▶

Week 14   Week 15   Week 16   Week 17

The Ultimate
POCKET
WORKOUT JOURNAL

BY ALEX A. LLUCH

HEALTH & FITNESS EXPERT AND
AUTHOR OF OVER 3 MILLION BOOKS SOLD!

THE ULTIMATE POCKET WORKOUT JOURNAL

BY ALEX A. LLUCH

Published by WS Publishing Group
San Diego, California 92119
Copyright © 2009 by WS Publishing Group

Fitness guidelines based on information provided by the United States Food and Drug Administration, Food and Nutrition Information Center, National Agricultural Library, Agricultural Research Service, and the U.S. Department of Agriculture.

Cover Image: ©iStockphoto/Beverley Vycital

Designed by WS Publishing Group:
David Defenbaugh

For inquiries:
Log on to www.WSPublishingGroup.com
E-mail info@WSPublishingGroup.com

ISBN-13: 978-1-934386-33-0

Printed in China

DISCLAIMER: The content in this book is provided for general informational purposes only and is not meant to substitute the advice provided by a medical professional. This information is not intended to diagnose or treat medical problems or substitute for appropriate medical care. If you are under the care of a physician and/or take medications for diabetes, heart disease, hypertension, or any other condition, consult your health care provider prior to initiation of any dietary program. Implementation of a dietary program may require altercation in your medication needs and must be done by or under the direction of your physician. If you have or suspect that you have a medical problem, promptly contact your health care provider. Never disregard professional medical advice or delay in seeking it because of something you have read in this book.

WS Publishing Group makes no claims whatsoever regarding the interpretation or utilization of any information contained herein and/or recorded by the user of this journal. If you utilize any information provided in this book, you do so at your own risk and you specifically waive any right to make any claim against the author and publisher, its officers, directors, employees or representatives as the result of the use of such information. Consult your physician before making any changes in your diet or exercise.

TABLE OF CONTENTS

INTRODUCTION.. 5
- What Is This Book About?.................................... 5
- Who Should Read This Book? 6
- What Is In This Book? 7

BENEFITING FROM BEING FIT 9
- Health Benefits.. 10
- Physical Benefits... 11
- Psychological Benefits... 13
- Additional Benefits of Physical Activity.......... 14

YOUR CURRENT FITNESS LEVEL 15
- Assessing Your Current Fitness Level 15
- Heart Rate.. 16
- Blood Pressure.. 18
- Body Composition.. 20
- Strength.. 24
- Flexibility... 28
- Fitness Test Results Worksheet 30

GETTING AND STAYING FIT!...................................... 31
- Setting Realistic Goals 32
- Creating a Plan 33
- Keeping Track of Your Progress 34
- Celebrating Achievements 35
- Helpful Hints for Getting and Staying Fit 36
- Adjusting Attitudes Toward Fitness.................. 37

CALORIES AND PHYSICAL ACTIVITIES 39

WATER AND FITNESS 43
- The Importance of Water and Fluids................. 43
- When to Drink 43

TABLE OF CONTENTS

- Sources of Hydration 44
- Hydration Before, During and After Your Workout 45
- Dehydration and Poor Performance 46

YOUR FITNESS PROFILE **47**
- Your Personal Health Profile Worksheet 47
- Physical Activity Readiness Questionnaire 48
- Fitness History 49

YOUR FITNESS GOALS **51**
- Fitness Preferences 51
- Workout Plan Questionnaire 52
- Exercise Excuses/Solutions Table 55

YOUR WORKOUT SCHEDULE **57**
- Your Workout Program Worksheet 59
- Tracking Your Results Worksheet 62
- Photo Progress Page 64

USING THE WORKOUT JOURNAL PAGES **65**
- Getting Started 65
- Cardiovascular Exercise 65
- Strength Training 66
- Flexibility, Relaxation, Meditation 66
- Water Intake 66
- Vitamins and Supplements 67
- Energy Level 67
- Calories Burned 67
- Notes/Reminders 68
- End-of-the-Week Wrap-Up 68

WORKOUT JOURNAL PAGES (WEEKS 1 THROUGH 26) **70**

INTRODUCTION

Getting fit will help you live a long, healthy, and enjoyable life. You don't have to live at the gym or make radical changes in your lifestyle. The benefits of getting fit are many, such as physical well-being, reduced stress, better sleep, increased self-esteem and greater self-confidence. With a combination of regular exercise and sensible eating, you will feel stronger, have greater endurance, and more energy.

It is true that becoming fit will involve commitment on your part. You will need to set aside some time each day to improve your physical conditioning and make healthy eating a priority. By reading this book you will find that getting fit can be fun and enjoyable. You will find by using the information contained in this book, getting fit is easier than you think.

WHAT IS THIS BOOK ABOUT?

This book will guide you through the basic principles of fitness and then teach you how to integrate them into your daily life. By encouraging you to examine your current fitness level and identify your personal goals, this book will help you create a personalized workout routine that you will follow and even enjoy.

This book is not a list of instructions that must be followed to the letter, but rather information and a journal that will accompany you on your journey to a new and healthier you. There are no get-fit-quick remedies in these pages. Instead,

INTRODUCTION

you will find real information that will help you make lasting changes to your lifestyle. Using the journal, you will plan your exercise routine and record your successes as you work toward a healthier and more satisfying lifestyle.

The pages that follow will also help you change the way you think about fitness. This book throws out the "no pain, no gain" and "do-or-die" attitudes and teaches you to view getting fit as a process that should be enjoyed. It will help you shift away from unrealistic media-driven expectations regarding fitness. This book will encourage you to adopt a more personal view of fitness that is based primarily on the effort you put forth. You will also discover how your success in getting fit will spill over into all aspects of your life.

WHO SHOULD READ THIS BOOK?

This book is for anyone who wants to learn how to get and stay fit. No matter what your age, this book will show you how anyone can improve their quality of life by adding regular physical exercise to their daily routine.

Parents should read this book, not only for themselves, but to be a good models for their children. Your children look up to you and learn from your actions. By showing them that fitness is an important aspect of your life, you will teach them to respect their own bodies and to make the right choices to stay fit and healthy.

INTRODUCTION
. . . .

WHAT IS IN THIS BOOK?

This book contains several special features, including the daily workout journal pages. Each section focuses on a specific aspect of physical fitness. Sections are arranged in a linear progression from baseline evaluation to creating your own personalized fitness routine.

Your Current Fitness Level and Getting and Staying Fit! provides simple methods for you to evaluate your current fitness level. This section will help you identify realistic fitness goals and develop a plan to achieve these goals by changing your attitude toward fitness and using helpful tips.

Calories and Physical Activities focuses on how the nutrients you eat and your caloric intake work in conjunction with the components of a complete exercise program to help you lose weight and get fit.

Water and Fitness evaluates the role proper hydration plays in your physical health. You will learn how your water intake can affect your physical performance and how adequate hydration can dramatically improve fitness.

Your Fitness Profile, Your Fitness Goals, and Your Workout Schedule provides a series of worksheets and tables to help you assess your current status and readiness for physical activities to better develop your fitness goals. You will record your goals in this section, as well as create a schedule for fitness. This section is designed to get you motivated and to keep you motivated throughout your fitness program. You will also record your results in this section, including pasting

INTRODUCTION

"Before" and "After" photos, which is a great way to visually assess your progress.

Workout Progress Chart will allow you to keep track of your progress. You can record your measurements, evaluate your results, and then set new goals as your fitness levels improve.

Workout Journal Pages are where you can keep a detailed record of your daily workouts. You can note your daily weight, the exercises you completed, your fluid intake, vitamins and supplements, and energy levels. Every page has space available for you to write down notes and reminders. End-of-the-Week Wrap-Up pages allow you to assess how you feel and what you accomplished for the entire week, as well as plan goals for the upcoming week.

This book presents a fresh perspective on health and fitness. It is designed to give you the tools to get fit and help you maintain your motivation throughout the process. Finally, the book will give you all the confidence you'll need to achieve your fitness goals.

BENEFITING FROM BEING FIT

What motivates people to get and stay fit? Why should people spend time, money and energy working out and being physically active when today's society is filled with more responsibilities and less time to accomplish them than ever before?

It's no surprise that over 60 percent of adults in the U.S. do not get the recommended amount of daily physical activity. Our long work hours, advances in modern technology, and increasing demands of our daily lives have led to a more sedentary lifestyle. In addition, the rise of fast food consumption and the availability of convenience foods have caused us to develop unhealthy eating habits. Our demanding work schedules, poor fitness and dietary habits have led Americans to become among the most obese and stressed people in the world.

In the past you may have not fully understood the benefits of daily physical activity or the consequences of a sedentary lifestyle. Or you may not have been able to overcome the obstacles that prevented you from working out. Maybe you did not know how to establish good habits that would enable you to stick with a physical fitness program. This time, with the information provided in this book combined with your commitment, you will get fit, feel great and enjoy a better quality of life.

Fitness is a choice you can make. You can decide to take the stairs versus the elevator, go to the gym instead of watching television, and wake up early and go for a run instead of sleeping in. Since you have purchased this book, you have probably already chosen to improve your physical fitness. You most likely have your own reasons for making that choice. You may have decided that you want to fit into a new pair of jeans; perhaps you've decided to run a marathon and need to get in shape; or maybe you've simply decided to lead a healthier lifestyle. Regardless of your motives, there are many valid and scientifically proven benefits of working out.

HEALTH BENEFITS

Research regarding the relationship between fitness and health is extensive and has been ongoing for decades. The results are clear: You will live longer if you are physically active. A Surgeon General's report on the benefits of physical activity concludes that even moderate exercise can substantially reduce the risk of developing or dying from diabetes, colon cancer and obesity-related illnesses.

Not being physically active can actually increase your risk of certain diseases. People who don't exercise are almost twice as likely to develop heart disease, which is the leading cause of death in the U.S.. Health experts say that millions of individuals in America suffer from many other chronic diseases that can be prevented through exercise. Clearly, it is in your best interest to be physically active.

BENEFITING FROM BEING FIT

Participating in a daily workout routine can benefit your health, just as inactivity can harm it. Scientific research conclusively proves that exercise helps lower cholesterol, reduce blood pressure, and prevent osteoporosis. Ongoing research is also providing evidence that exercise also protects against arthritis, certain kinds of cancer, and numerous other diseases.

PHYSICAL BENEFITS

The physical effects of exercise can be extremely gratifying. There are three main benefits that you will experience when you incorporate a workout into your daily routine. First, you will experience an overall improvement in your physical appearance as you increase lean muscle mass, lose weight, and gain strength. Second, you will benefit from an increased metabolism as your body becomes more efficient at burning food for energy. In addition, you will feel more rested and have more energy because you will experience improved sleep.

How exercise achieves these benefits is not mysterious. For example, a daily exercise program can help you look better by allowing you to control your weight and build muscle mass. Without exercise, muscle mass decreases and body fat increases. When you work out on a regular basis, the body becomes more defined, toned and athletic. The process of gaining muscle mass occurs when a muscle is repeatedly activated against some form of resistance, such as when you lift weights. In response to this exertion, a muscle will grow larger and stronger in order to

. . . .

fulfill this new physical demand.

Increasing your lean muscle mass actually increases your ability to burn fat. Muscles consume more calories than other types of tissues do. You can burn approximately 50 more calories a day for every pound of added muscle. A regular workout routine, combined with a sensible diet, allows the body to use more calories than it is ingesting. This forces the body to convert stored fat into energy. Body weight decreases and you become stronger, leaner, and more defined. Clothes fit better. You stand taller and straighter, since stronger muscles help improve your posture; overall you look and feel more confident.

One of the many physical benefits of exercise is an improved metabolism. Metabolism refers to the amount of calories your body burns to stay alive. Specifically, it refers to the speed and efficiency with which the body is able to break down food and convert it into energy. Regular exercise helps facilitate the body's ability to burn calories by maximizing the flow of oxygen-laden blood throughout the body. The more oxygen your body receives, the more calories you burn.

Regular exercise is one way to foster healthy sleep. The body has a natural cycle in which it alternates between states of inactivity during sleep and arousal while awake. These cycles are symbiotic, meaning that they depend on one another. If the body remains too sedentary during its active phase, it may have a difficult transition into its sleep phase. However, if the body is forced to work and intensify its active period, it will conversely enter into a deeper rest period. Tests have shown that those who maintain a regular exercise routine benefit from a more consistent and restful sleep. Increased sleep results in an improvement in vitality, mental acuity and mood.

PSYCHOLOGICAL BENEFITS

The psychological improvements that result through regular exercise are just as abundant and transforming as the health and physical benefits. Evidence shows that those who exercise moderately on a regular basis have lower levels of anxiety and are less likely to suffer from depression. Routine exercisers also report increased self-esteem and overall happiness. These feelings are most intense for a few hours after exercise due to the release of naturally occurring substances, called endorphins, into the bloodstream. Endorphins relax muscles and give a person an overall feeling of relaxation and contentment. Research suggests that as the body increases its ability to exercise it also increases its ability to produce endorphins. Consequently, more exercise leads to feeling better longer.

Maintaining a fitness routine creates a feeling of accomplishment and confidence. Many people find that success in transforming themselves physically has a collateral effect in other aspects of their lives. For example, increased confidence and self-esteem can enhance your ability in your professional and social life.

BENEFITING FROM BEING FIT

....

ADDITIONAL BENEFITS OF PHYSICAL ACTIVITY

The combined health, physical and psychological benefits of physical fitness foster an overall lifestyle change. With increased energy and self-confidence, new opportunities are opened. Whereas a sedentary lifestyle is limiting, a healthy, fit lifestyle expands your horizons. Many people find that increased self-confidence and energy can lead to an increased desire to engage in new social and physical activities. The end result is an improvement in one's overall quality of life.

People who maintain a regular physical fitness routine find an increased desire to engage in new physical activities. Increased energy allows individuals to pursue new activities that were hindered by their previous sedentary lifestyle. People who maintain a regular fitness routine are more able to pursue activities that they find personally satisfying. For example, those who enjoy nature have renewed energy to take hikes and bicycle rides. Those who enjoy sports are able to play and compete at a more competitive level.

An active lifestyle increases opportunities to make new friends. Exercise itself may become the source of social interactions. Whether in the form of casual conversation with others in the gym or by joining an organized class, exercise is an excellent way to make friends or develop new interests. While classic forms of exercise like team sports and spinning (bicycling) classes continue to be popular, alternative forms like ballroom dancing and yoga have also gained new interest and availability.

YOUR CURRENT FITNESS LEVEL

Each individual has his or her unique potential for physical fitness based on the interaction of genetics, health status and lifestyle. Therefore, the first step in getting fit is determining your current physical condition. This information will be used to establish your baseline level of fitness. This chapter contains a series of simple tests used to quantify your starting point on the road to fitness. These tests will focus on cardiovascular health, body composition, strength and flexibility. The information provided in this section can be used as a guide to systematically tailor an exercise plan to reach your personal fitness goals.

Record the results of these tests on the Fitness Test Results Worksheet on page 30. In later chapters, these numbers will be used to prepare realistic fitness goals and track personal progress and success.

Important reminder: A doctor should be consulted before beginning any rigorous exercise program. This is especially important if you are taking medication for high blood pressure or are being treated for any other physical condition.

ASSESSING YOUR CURRENT FITNESS LEVEL

Begin by assessing your current fitness level. Use this assessment to create a realistic fitness plan. This baseline assessment includes attention to (1) heart rate, (2) blood pressure, (3) body composition, (4) strength, and (5) flexibility.

HEART RATE

The heart rate is a leading indicator of your baseline fitness level and can be used as a guide to maximize the results of cardiovascular exercise. The heart is a specialized muscle that is designed to pump the blood needed to maintain all of your bodily functions. Blood brings oxygen and nutrients to every part of the body. A heart's performance is essential to sustaining life all the way down to the cellular level.

Your heart rate is the number of times your heart beats in a minute. This number is a clear indicator of the strength of your heart. A strong heart pumps more effectively with each contraction and therefore doesn't need to beat as fast to supply the body with blood. A high heart rate indicates that the heart is not as efficient at circulating blood and therefore needs to pump faster to keep up with your body's needs. As your heart becomes better at pumping blood through regular exercise, you will find that your heart rate will decrease. Find your resting and active heart rates by following the simple instructions below. Use these numbers to determine your current fitness level.

A resting heart rate is simply the number of times the heart beats in a minute when you're not moving around. It is important that you sit or lie down and remain motionless for at least

YOUR CURRENT FITNESS LEVEL

. . . .

, minutes before making this measurement. Once you're completely relaxed, place 2 fingers against the inside of the wrist or alongside the neck. Count the number of beats for 15 seconds and then multiply that number by 4. Record this figure in the Fitness Test Results Worksheet on page 30. Compare your heart rate to the table, which provides heart rate fitness levels by age and gender.

Resting Heart Rate Fitness by Age and Gender

MEN BY AGE GROUP

RESTING HEART RATE	AGE IN YEARS					
	18–25	26–35	36–45	46–55	56–65	65+
EXCELLENT	50–60	50–61	51–62	51–63	52–61	51–61
GOOD	61–68	62–69	63–69	64–70	62–70	62–68
AVERAGE	69–76	70–77	70–78	71–79	71–78	69–75
FAIR	77-80	78-80	79-81	80-83	79-80	76-78
POOR	81+	81+	82+	84+	81+	79+

WOMEN BY AGE GROUP

RESTING HEART RATE	AGE IN YEARS					
	18–25	26–35	36–45	46–55	56–65	65+
EXCELLENT	55–64	55–63	55–63	55–64	55–63	55–63
GOOD	65–72	64–71	64–72	65–72	64–72	64–71
AVERAGE	73–80	72–78	73–80	73–79	73–79	72–79
FAIR	81-83	79-81	81-83	80-82	80-82	80-81
POOR	84+	82+	84+	83+	83+	82+

Fitness can also be evaluated in terms of what is called your active heart rate. An active heart rate indicates your heart's maximum potential or ability to work under strain. An active heart rate is important for measuring improvement in your fitness, specifically with regard to aerobic fitness.

BLOOD PRESSURE

It is important to determine your blood pressure before starting a physical fitness program. Those suffering from high blood pressure should contact a medical professional before beginning any physical fitness routine. Blood pressure is the force of blood against the arteries and is created by the heart as it pumps blood through the circulatory system. Like all muscles, the heart cycles between contracting and relaxing; blood pressure varies accordingly. Systolic blood pressure refers to the pressure when the heart contracts. Diastolic pressure refers to the pressure when the heart relaxes. Blood pressure is expressed by these two figures, with the systolic reading listed over the diastolic figure (e.g., 130/90).

Many pharmacies are equipped with machines that allow customers to measure their own blood pressure. This may serve as a quick way to generally measure baseline blood pressure, but a trained professional can give you the most reliable reading. When you're visiting your doctor in advance of beginning an exercise program, your blood pressure will certainly be checked and recorded. Write your blood pressure on the Fitness Test

YOUR CURRENT FITNESS LEVEL

Results Worksheet on page 30. Compare your blood pressure to the table on the following page, which lists blood pressure figures and their corresponding risk categories.

Individuals who are overweight often suffer from high blood pressure, or hypertension. Hypertension is dangerous because it strains the heart as it pumps blood through the body. Over time, the strain can lead to heart muscle breakdown and deterioration. This leaves the heart weakened and increases the chance of a heart attack, stroke, and heart failure. In addition, hypertension can lead to chronic kidney failure.

Blood Pressure and Corresponding Risk Level

SYSTOLIC	DIASTOLIC	STAGE AND HEALTH RISK
210	120	High Blood Pressure • Hypertension Stage 4 • Very Severe Risk
180	110	High Blood Pressure • Hypertension Stage 3 • Severe
160	100	High Blood Pressure • Hypertension Stage 2 • Moderate Risk
140	90	High Blood Pressure • Hypertension Stage 1 • Mild Risk
140	90	Borderline High
130	90	High Normal
120	85	Normal • Optimum
110	75	Low Normal
90	60	Borderline Low
60	40	Low Blood Pressure • Hypotension
50	33	Very Low Blood Pressure • Extreme Danger

YOUR CURRENT FITNESS LEVEL

BODY COMPOSITION

The body functions best when it consists of a proper proportion of muscle, fat, organs and bone. Your body composition is determined by the ratio of these elements against the body's mass. While bone and organs' mass and weight remain relatively constant, everyone's fat and muscle weight varies. The percent of body weight that is made up of fat and muscle is an important indicator of body composition and overall fitness. Without proper amounts of both muscle and fat, the body will fail to work at its optimum level.

A person who appears thin may still have a high fat percentage and therefore be unhealthy. People who undergo crash or extreme diets will often lose more muscle mass than fat. If you try to lose weight by dieting without exercising, lean muscle mass may decrease, resulting in an increased fat percentage. Exercise will keep that from happening. Regular exercise forces muscles to engage and work to exhaustion. This, coupled with adequate rest, forces your muscles to adapt by growing larger and stronger. The increased muscle mass diminishes your body's fat percentage and increases its overall health.

Fat is essential to many functions of the body. However, excess fat, especially in the waist area, puts you at increased risk of cardiovascular disease and other health problems such as heart attacks, strokes, and diabetes. In addition, new research shows a correlation between most forms of cancer (except skin cancer) and excess body fat. While genetic predispositions and

. . . .

environmental factors can put you at risk of developing cancer and many other diseases, excess weight increases these risks by making it more difficult for the body to fight off infection and rebuild damaged tissues.

Body composition and fat percentages can be determined in numerous ways:

Hydrostatic Weighing: The most accurate method of measuring body composition is called hydrostatic weighing. This involves weighing a person in air and then again while submerged in water. However accurate this method might be, it is not very practical due to the specialized equipment needed and the complexity of the procedure.

Bioelectrical Impedance Analysis (BIA): The BIA is a computerized examination that helps medical professionals determine the specific composition of the body, including its fat percentage. This is a noninvasive test administered by a doctor and takes about ten minutes. A BIA can also detect the presence of disease, nutrient and water deficiency, environmental and industrial pollutants, oxidative damage and other ailments. With this information a health care provider can create a fitness and diet routine that helps correct a variety of conditions.

Caliper Test: The most common and relatively accurate method for measuring body fat is what's known as a skin fold, or caliper, test. Using a specialized instrument called a caliper, the person conducting the test pinches folds of skin on various locations throughout the body. This test is available at many gyms or fitness facilities.

Body Mass Index (BMI): Less accurate than hydrostatic weighing or a caliper skin fold test, the BMI uses a person's height and weight to determine an approximate fat percentage. Healthcare professionals often use a person's BMI to determine his or her cardiovascular health risk. While all bodies are different, they all generally conform to this scale. While each person's frame varies, the range provided in the BMI takes that into consideration. Your BMI can be determined by taking your weight (in kilograms) and dividing it by its height (in meters) squared; the formula is simple: $Kg/m2 = BMI$. Your approximate BMI can be found using your body's height (feet) and weight (lbs) in the following table. This table also shows the cardiovascular risks associated with various ranges of BMI readings.

YOUR CURRENT FITNESS LEVEL

Body Mass Index (BMI) and Cardiovascular Risk Chart for Men and Women

BMI	19	20	21	22	23	24	25	26	27	28	29	30	31	32	33	34	35
Height								Weight in pounds									
4'10"	91	96	100	105	110	115	119	124	129	134	138	143	148	153	158	162	167
4'11"	94	99	104	109	114	119	124	128	133	138	143	148	153	158	163	168	173
5'	97	102	107	112	118	123	128	133	138	143	148	153	158	163	158	174	179
5'1"	100	106	111	116	122	127	132	137	143	148	153	158	164	169	174	180	185
5'2"	104	109	115	120	126	131	136	142	147	153	158	164	169	175	180	186	191
5'3"	107	113	118	124	130	135	141	146	152	158	163	169	175	180	186	191	197
5'4"	110	116	122	128	134	140	145	151	157	163	169	174	180	186	192	197	204
5'5"	114	120	126	132	138	144	150	156	162	168	174	180	186	192	198	204	210
5'6"	118	124	130	136	142	148	155	161	167	173	179	186	192	198	204	210	216
5'7"	121	127	134	140	146	153	159	166	172	178	185	191	198	204	211	217	223
5'8"	125	131	138	144	151	158	164	171	177	184	190	197	203	210	216	223	230
5'9"	128	135	142	149	155	162	169	176	182	189	196	203	209	216	223	230	236
5'10"	132	139	146	153	160	167	174	181	188	195	202	209	216	222	229	236	243
5'11"	136	143	150	157	165	172	179	186	193	200	208	215	222	229	236	243	250
6'	140	147	154	162	169	177	184	191	199	206	213	221	228	235	242	250	258
6'1"	144	151	159	166	174	182	189	197	204	212	219	227	235	242	250	257	265
6'2"	148	155	163	171	179	186	194	202	210	218	225	233	241	249	256	264	272
6'3"	152	160	168	176	184	192	200	208	216	224	232	240	248	256	264	272	279

| Healthy | Overweight | Obese |

Record your approximate BMI on the Fitness Test Results Worksheet on page 30.

YOUR CURRENT FITNESS LEVEL

STRENGTH

Your body's physical strength shows the condition of your muscles and their ability to function at maximum output. Strength is the amount of force a muscle can produce. It can be measured in the amount of weight the muscle can lift or how much force it can exert as you jump, hit a golf ball, or engage in other activities. By measuring your muscles' strength you can get a sense of your overall fitness. This measurement can help you create a fitness plan and measure future successes. Follow the instructions for each of the following strength tests and record the results in the Fitness Results Worksheet on page 30.

Push-up Test: This test focuses on the strength and endurance of muscles in your upper body. Gently stretch and warm up your arm, chest and shoulder muscles. Avoid over-exertion in order to get the most accurate test results. Men should assume the traditional push-up position, with only the hands and tips of the toes touching the ground. Women should assume the bent knee position, with knees and hands touching the ground. No matter which position you use, you should keep the head, neck and back aligned. Start by bending your arms and slowly lowering your chest until it's four inches from the ground, keeping your back and legs straight. Then straighten the arms and push your body back into the starting position. Be sure not to lock your elbows. The back and legs should remain straight and the head and neck in line at all times. Repeat this as many times as you can while maintaining proper form. Count the number of

YOUR CURRENT FITNESS LEVEL

repetitions before fatigue forces you to stop.

Record the number in the Fitness Test Results Worksheet on page 30. The following table will help you estimate your condition based on your age, gender, and the number of push-ups you can do.

Push-up Fitness for Men

NO. OF PUSH-UPS	MEN'S AGE					
	13-19	20's	30's	40's	50's	60's
Excellent	45+	40+	35+	29+	25+	23+
Good	31-41	26-35	22-29	18-25	15-22	14-20
Average	26-29	26-35	18-21	15-17	12-14	10-13
Fair	14-24	12-21	9-17	7-14	5-11	3-9
Poor	14-	12-	9-	7-	5-	3-

Push-up Fitness for Women

NO. OF PUSH-UPS	WOMEN'S AGE					
	13-19	20's	30's	40's	50's	60's
Excellent	32+	30+	28+	24+	20+	18+
Good	21-28	19-26	18-26	15-22	12-18	11-16
Average	17-20	16-18	14-17	12-14	10-12	8-10
Fair	9-16	8-15	5-13	4-11	3-9	2-7
Poor	8-	7-	4-	3-	2-	1-

YOUR CURRENT FITNESS LEVEL

Sit up-Test: The sit-up test assesses your abdominal muscles' fitness and stamina. Lie on the floor, facing up with knees bent and place your feet shoulder-width apart. Start by pressing your lower back into the ground and place your arms across your chest. Lift your head, neck and shoulders off the floor and bring your body into a sitting position by engaging the stomach muscles. The abdomen should be contracted as your upper body is brought to a 90-degree angle with the floor. Then slowly roll back down into the starting position while keeping the abdominal muscles tight.

Record the number of repetitions per minute in the Fitness Test Results Worksheet on page 30 and compare your number with the following chart.

One Minute Sit-up Test for Men

| | MEN'S AGE | | | | | |
	18-25	26-35	36-45	46-55	56-65	65+
Excellent	32+	30+	28+	24+	20+	18+
Good	21–28	19–26	18–26	15–22	12–18	11–16
Average	17–20	16–18	14–17	12–14	10–12	8–10
Fair	9–16	8–15	5–13	4–11	3–9	2–7
Poor	8-	7-	4-	3-	2-	1-

NO. OF SIT-UPS

YOUR CURRENT FITNESS LEVEL

One Minute Sit-up Test for Women

		WOMEN'S AGE				
		18-25	26-35	36-45	46-55	56-65	65+
Excellent		43+	39+	33+	27 +	24+	23+
Good		35–42	31–38	25–32	20–26	16–23	15–22
Average		28–34	24–30	18–24	13–19	9–15	10–14
Fair		23–27	19–23	14–17	9–12	6–8	4–9
Poor		22-	18-	13-	8-	5-	3-

(NO. OF SIT-UPS)

Squat Test: The Squat test focuses on the strength of the lower body. Stand up straight with your feet shoulder-width apart. Just as if you are sitting back into a chair, bring your hips back and lower your body until your upper legs are parallel to the floor. Keep your knees and heels aligned at all times. With your head and chest lifted, return to a standing position. A chair may be placed underneath as a guide, but must not be used to rest in between squats. Count how many squats are completed before you tire and must stop.

Record the number in the Fitness Test Result Worksheet on page 30 and compare your number with the following chart.

YOUR CURRENT FITNESS LEVEL

Squats Fitness Determined by Age

			WOMEN'S AGE			
		18-25	26-35	36-45	46-55	56-65	65+
Excellent		49+	45+	41+	35+	31+	28+
Good		40-48	36-44	31-40	26-34	22-30	20-27
Average	NO. OF SIT-UPS	35-39	31-35	27-30	22-25	17-21	15-19
Fair		29-34	27-30	21-26	16-21	12-16	10-14
Poor		28-	26-	20-	15-	11-	9-

FLEXIBILITY

The most commonly overlooked aspect of physical fitness is flexibility. Flexibility is the range of motion of the body's joints. Flexibility is the result of muscles, tendons and ligaments working together. People will often focus on increasing their body's muscles without taking flexibility into consideration. As muscle strength increases, the body exerts more force on the tendons and ligaments. It's important, therefore, to increase your flexibility so as to avoid injury to tendons and ligaments. You can become more flexible by stretching. Stretching should be approached with the same care and precision that you would bring to any other aspect of an exercise routine. Incorporate stretching into every workout. With increased flexibility you will be more able to increase your strength and endurance while decreasing the chance of injury. Without proper stretching, these crucial tissues can be damaged under the new strain. Stretching enables the tendons and ligaments to handle the stress and grow with the muscles.

YOUR CURRENT FITNESS LEVEL

Sit and Reach Test: The sit and reach test measures the flexibility of your hamstrings and lower back. Before you begin, make sure you warm up. Place a ruler or tape measure on the floor with the numbers increasing away from you. Sit on the floor with your legs straight so that your heels line up with the 23-inch mark. The numbers should get higher past your heels. While seated, place your hands on top of each other and stretch forward toward your toes without bouncing. Slowly reach three times and on the fourth reach record your measurement. Have someone stand over you as you reach so they can read the stretch correctly for you. The numbers listed in the table below offer median measurements. Age and arm length contribute to scoring differences.

Record results in the Fitness Test Results Worksheet on page 30 and compare your number with the following chart.

Sit & Reach Flexibility

	SUPERIOR	EXCELLENT	GOOD	AVERAGE	POOR
MEN	27"+	25-27"	23-25"	21-23"	< 20"
WOMEN	30"+	28-30"	26-28"	24-26"	< 23"

YOUR CURRENT FITNESS LEVEL

FITNESS TEST RESULTS WORKSHEET

Use the following worksheet to record the results of the tests taken in this chapter. These numbers will be used in later chapters to prepare a fitness routine with realistic and achievable goals.

DATE: ___ / ___ / ___

TEST	INITIAL	3 MONTHS	6 MONTHS	9 MONTHS	12 MONTHS
HEART RATE (RESTING)					
BLOOD PRESSURE					
BODY FAT %					
BODY MASS INDEX					
PUSH-UP					
SIT-UP					
SQUAT					
SIT & REACH					

GETTING AND STAYING FIT!

There are four keys to success when creating and maintaining a workout program: (1) Setting Realistic Goals, (2) Creating a Plan, (3) Keeping Track of Progress, and (4) Celebrating Achievement. Together, they will help change your lifestyle and alter your views about working out.

While each person has a different motivation for getting fit, the reasons an exercise routine fails are usually the same: burnout, injury, or failure to meet goals. Focusing on the positive aspects of working out is crucial to overcoming the mental obstacles that are common among people in any fitness program. Concentrating on the benefits you will gain from your routine is important. If you can see the evidence of your achievements, you are more likely to maintain your efforts to attain your personal fitness goals.

The way you perceive working out can impact the success of your program. Try to maintain a positive attitude during your workout program. It is important to avoid the negativity that can result if you deviate from your plan. It is very common for people just starting out to become frustrated if they don't see immediate progress or if they have to miss a session. It is important to combat negative thoughts such as "My day is ruined" by remembering that an occasional missed session is insignificant in the context of a long-term fitness routine. A missed session can be an excellent motivational tool. Refocus your energy and determination during your next workout session.

GETTING AND STAYING FIT!

Recognize that change takes time. The keys to maintaining a fitness routine are patience, consistency and discipline. Fitness should be an ongoing endeavor. During this journey, make sure you don't lose sight of the benefits of exercise. Enjoy the changes in your body, your better mood, and increased energy. Feel the sense of accomplishment when you take positive actions towards a healthier lifestyle. Fitness is not just a goal to be reached, but rather a new way to live.

SETTING REALISTIC GOALS

Many fitness routines fail or are abandoned because of unrealistic goals. Setting unrealistic goals can make it extremely difficult to keep up with a fitness routine. It is important to consider how you phrase your fitness and exercise goals. Statements like "I'm going to lose 20 pounds in 3 months" are unrealistic and will most likely result in failure. It is critical to replace the results-based statements (like the one above) with statements about the effort you plan to put forth toward realistic steps to achieve fitness goals (e.g., "I will work out 3 times a week for at least 30 minutes."). Individuals who set unrealistic goals might overexert themselves, resulting in burnout or injury. Or an individual will become discouraged after failing to meet an unrealistic expectation and give up on the routine. The bottom line is to establish a workout routine with achievable short-term and long-term goals.

By taking a realistic look at all of the factors that influence your physical fitness, you can begin to set realistic short- and long-term goals. Goals should be based on your body type, current physical condition, and life circumstances. General

. . . .

long-term goals can include weight loss, better endurance, or a more muscular physical appearance. Try to narrow down these broad goals so they are specific and measurable. If weight loss is a goal, determine your target weight or chose an article of clothing that you want to fit into. If you are looking to improve your endurance, make your goal completing a half-marathon. After you have determined your long-term goals, break them down into more immediate ones. Use these short-term goals to track your progress and measure the success of your program. Once a short-term goal is achieved, replace it with a new one. If progress towards a goal is slow, try changing your routine to see better results. Make sure your long-term and short-term goals are attainable, yet challenging. Goals can be both physical achievements, such as hiking to the top of a local mountain, or related to the fitness routine itself—for example, completing a workout session 3 times a week for 4 straight weeks.

CREATING A PLAN

Fitness plans that work best incorporate your likes and dislikes. It is important to choose a program that is appropriate for your lifestyle and ability. If you don't feel comfortable in a gym and prefer to work out alone, chose a routine that can be accomplished at home or at a local park. You're more likely to stick with a fitness routine molded to match your lifestyle.

While every plan should be created to meet the needs of the individual, all plans should include diversity and fun. A fitness plan should contain a variety of activities. This will help prevent boredom and injury. By varying the routine, the body is forced to adapt in new ways, making an injury from an unaccustomed move or exercise less likely.

All fitness plans should include a minimum of each of the three main types of fitness programs (strength, cardiovascular and flexibility). The body cannot achieve its maximum potential unless you attend to all three types of fitness programs together. Neglecting or eliminating one of these elements can result in fatigue, decreased performance, and injury.

KEEPING TRACK OF YOUR PROGRESS

It is important to keep track of your progress. Monitoring your progress on a regular basis with the workout journal in this book will help you stay motivated, focused and disciplined. It will also help you determine the effectiveness of your routine and measure your success. Everyone's body is different, therefore, progress will vary from one person to another.

Sometimes, it may even seem like you're losing ground, but that may not be cause for concern. For example, people will often gain weight initially when beginning a fitness routine. This happens due to the increase in muscle mass. This weight gain should not be interpreted as failure, but as an indicator that your body is changing. These types of changes are why continuous monitoring is critical.

If weight loss is the main goal of a fitness program, it is logical that weight is an important measure of progress. Weigh measurements should be done in the most uniform way possible. Each weighing should happen at roughly the same time of the day. For the most consistent and accurate results, weigh

GETTING AND STAYING FIT!

. . . .

yourself in the morning before getting dressed.

As mentioned earlier, it is also important to set and keep track of the immediate goals regarding the frequency, intensity, and duration of your workouts. For example, if you want to gain strength, you will need to weight train 2 or 3 times a week. In this case, it is important to record how often you work out, as well as the weight, repetitions and sets for each exercise. Use the daily workout journal included in this book to keep track of your fitness routine and to make notes regarding your progress. Keeping track of your fitness routine on a daily basis will help you recognize your achievements, stay motivated, and indicate when you need to modify your program.

CELEBRATING ACHIEVEMENTS

Years of research show that reinforcement is key to incorporating new behaviors (e.g., regularly going to the gym) into your life. Celebrating your achievements will increase the likelihood that you will continue with your fitness routine. Therefore, it is important to reward yourself when you make progress toward your short- and long-term goals.

Be sure to incorporate an incentive program into your fitness plan. Reward yourself only when you achieve a specific goal. For example, you might decide that going to the gym 3 times per week for 1 month deserves a reward. Achieving a certain level of weight loss might be another good milestone for earning a treat.

The type of reward you give yourself is just as important as the achievement you are celebrating. Rewards should be carefully selected to support your workout program. Rewards should be healthy and should not be something that you will obtain regardless of your results. For example, a vacation that you have already planned and paid for is not a good reward since you are going to get that whether or not you stick to your workout schedule. Instead, choose something that is extra, such as going to a movie, buying a new pair of shoes, or splurging on a massage.

HELPFUL HINTS FOR GETTING AND STAYING FIT

Here are some helpful tips for starting
and maintaining a fitness plan:

Schedule and plan your workouts in advance. Write down your program on a calendar a week ahead of time. Avoid saying things like, "If I have time, I'll go for a run." If you plan ahead you can fit workouts into a busy schedule.

Keep a positive attitude. Don't worry if you slip up on occasion and miss a session. Just use it as motivation to make the most of your next workout.

Start the day with exercise. Those who work out in the morning enjoy the effects all day long.

Find a "fitness buddy." Your partner should be someone who has similar fitness goals. Encouragement from friends can be very motivating.

GETTING AND STAYING FIT!

ADJUSTING ATTITUDES TOWARD FITNESS

Your attitude toward exercise is just as important as the exercise itself. The goal is to change the way you view exercise. Use the following techniques to change your mental outlook and increase the benefits of exercise.

Focus: When exercising, it is important to focus on the task at hand. Concentrating on your exercise will help you maximize the results you achieve during a session. Distraction often leads to boredom, which is one of the reasons people stop working out.

Visualization: Before beginning any fitness routine, it is helpful to attach some visual image to the routine. It is important to imagine the most specific images and sounds possible. For example, you might imagine the sound of lifting weights off the rack, and connect that image to arriving at the top of a mountain. Think about how a mountain's rocky terrain feels under your feet and how the spectacular view from the top makes you feel.

Realization: A successful workout routine is the result of willpower, determination, and the desire to accomplish your goals. As you make progress, you realize that you can achieve great things. Use this realization when you're fatigued, depressed, or bored. Knowing you have achieved something and realizing that you can do it even better the next time will lift your aspirations to new levels. Positive thinking will encourage you to persevere through moments of self-doubt and negativity.

Redirection: If you begin to doubt your abilities, simply redirect that negativity into something positive and believe in it. Replace every negative thought with a more powerful positive thought. For example, "I can't" becomes, "I've succeeded already. I can do it again!"

In the End-of-the-Week Wrap-Up sections of your journal, you can record changes in your mental outlook, along with your physical. You will find that your newfound confidence and positive mental outlook will transfer to other aspects of your life. People who regularly exercise often become more patient, resistant to discouragement, and enjoy a more positive outlook on life!

CALORIES AND PHYSICAL ACTIVITIES

We burn the calories that food provides in the course of exercising and in our daily activities. Even when we're sleeping, we burn some calories. The more vigorous the activity, the more calories we burn.

Depending on what kind of work we do or what activities we engage in at home, we may use up a lot of calories during the day. The table on the next page shows the amount of calories burned during typical daily activities. You can use this chart to calculate the approximate number of calories you burn in the course of a day. When you know how many calories you are expending each day, you can balance the number of calories you take in against the number of calories you burn. This information will help you make healthy choices when it comes to planning a diet.

For most of us, our jobs and other day-to-day activities don't involve enough exercise to use up the calories we get from the food we eat. Without regular exercise, we are likely to put on weight. That weight, unfortunately, will be in the form of fat. Refer to the table on the next page to determine the number of calories you can expect to burn for each hour of moderate and vigorous activity. If you incorporate moderate or vigorous exercise into your daily routine, you can expect not only to control your weight, but to become more fit.

CALORIES AND PHYSICAL ACTIVITIES

CALORIES BURNED FOR TYPICAL PHYSICAL ACTIVITIES

LIGHT ACTIVITIES: 150 or less	CAL/HR
Billiards	140
Lying down/sleeping	60
Office work	140
Sitting	80
Standing	100

MODERATE ACTIVITIES: 150-350	CAL/HR
Aerobic dancing	340
Ballroom dancing	210
Bicycling (5 mph)	170
Bowling	160
Canoeing (2.5 mph)	170
Dancing (social)	210
Gardening (moderate)	270
Golf (with cart)	180
Golf (without cart)	320
Grocery shopping	180
Horseback riding (sitting trot)	250
Light housework/cleaning, etc.	250
Ping-pong	270
Swimming (20 yards/min)	290
Tennis (recreational doubles)	310
Vacuuming	220
Volleyball (recreational)	260
Walking (2 mph)	200
Walking (3 mph)	240
Walking (4 mph)	300

CALORIES AND PHYSICAL ACTIVITIES

CALORIES BURNED FOR TYPICAL PHYSICAL ACTIVITIES

VIGOROUS ACTIVITIES: 350 or MORE   CAL/HR.

Aerobics (step)	440
Backpacking (10 lb load)	540
Badminton	450
Basketball (competitive)	660
Basketball (leisure)	390
Bicycling (10 mph)	375
Bicycling (13 mph)	600
Cross country skiing (leisurely)	460
Cross country skiing (moderate)	660
Hiking	460
Ice skating (9 mph)	384
Jogging (5 mph)	550
Jogging (6 mph)	690
Racquetball	620
Rollerblading	384
Rowing machine	540
Running (8 mph)	900
Scuba diving	570
Shoveling snow	580
Soccer	580
Spinning	650
Stair climber machine	480
Swimming (50 yards/min.)	680
Water aerobics	400
Water skiing	480
Weight training (30 sec. between sets)	760
Weight training (60 sec. between sets)	570

NOTES

WATER AND FITNESS

Water is essential to survival. Water constitutes more than two-thirds of the human body. In addition, water is crucial to all of your body's major functions. Without enough water, you cannot digest food or eliminate wastes properly. Deprived of water, your body will quickly shut down.

THE IMPORTANCE OF WATER AND FLUIDS

Drinking enough water is crucial if we are to perform our day-to-day tasks effectively. When you do not have enough water, symptoms of dehydration quickly develop. Signs of dehydration include headaches, difficulty concentrating, and fatigue. Under such conditions, being effective at work or at home becomes difficult or impossible.

The consequences of dehydration are serious. Prolonged dehydration can increase the risk of kidney stones, infections and other serious health problems. On the other hand, maintaining hydration can have tremendous benefits. Recent studies have shown that people who drink at least 8 glasses of water a day can decrease their risk of developing colon, bladder, and even breast cancer.

WHEN TO DRINK

As important as staying well hydrated is, it's easy to forget to drink water until dehydration has already set in. Research has shown that the best time to drink water is before you feel thirsty. Physical signs like dry mouth and sensations of thirst often occur only after you are dehydrated.

Even when people remember to drink water, they often fail to drink enough. The amount of water required for each individual is determined by his or her weight and metabolism. A rule of thumb for calculating your water consumption needs is to take your weight in pounds and divide it in half. The resulting number is the number of ounces of water you should consume. For example, a 180-pound person should drink 90 ounces of water per day. Some experts, however, suggest drinking even more water. They say that on average, men should drink around 120 ounces of water per day, while women should have around 90 ounces. No matter what your ideal water consumption is, remember to increase your water intake in conditions such as high heat, high altitude, low humidity, or high activity level.

SOURCES OF HYDRATION

A number of liquids and solid foods can provide your body with the water it needs:

Water: Your body uses water most readily in its plain, unadulterated form. The bulk (80 to 90 percent) of your hydration should come from drinking plain water.

Beverages: Drinking non-caffeinated beverages such as fruit juices, sports drinks, and milk is a good way of maintaining your hydration. Herbal teas also work well. Just remember that many beverages also contain sugar, fat, or both, which can add unwanted calories to your diet.

Fruits and vegetables: These solid foods consist mainly of water and therefore are excellent for hydration. Individuals who eat a healthy amount of fruits and vegetables may receive up to 20 percent of their hydration from these solid foods.

Be wary of drinking caffeinated beverages, such as coffee, tea and many soft drinks. Caffeine is a diuretic, meaning that it stimulates your kidneys to remove water from your system. If you feel the need for a caffeinated beverage, remember to compensate by drinking extra water.

HYDRATION BEFORE, DURING AND AFTER YOUR WORKOUT

Proper hydration is one of the easiest and most effective ways of boosting workout performance. Water is necessary in order for metabolism to take place, so being properly hydrated helps your body turn food into the energy you need for exercising. Water also helps your body regulate its temperature through sweating. Because vigorous exercise causes you to lose large amounts of water through sweating, it is important to drink water before, during, and after each workout session.

Pre-workout: Drink between 8 and 16 ounces of water in the hour prior to working out.

During workout: Replenish fluids by drinking 4 to 8 ounces of water every fifteen minutes. During vigorous cardiovascular training, or if you're exercising in hot temperatures, increase your water consumption in order to replace water lost from sweating.

After workout: Drink between 8 and 16 ounces of water within thirty minutes of completing your exercise routine. Your muscles need water in order to recover from the stress of a workout. Drinking proper amounts of water after your workout will help reduce muscle soreness and help you feel less tired.

Experts say that if your goal is to lose weight, you should increase the amount of water you consume before and after working out. Water is necessary for metabolism to take place. By keeping well hydrated, you will help your body burn calories.

DEHYDRATION AND POOR PERFORMANCE

Just as keeping hydrated enhances physical performance, dehydration leads to decreases in physical and mental performance. When you are dehydrated your body is unable to handle the physical exertions related to cardiovascular or strength exercises. As you become dehydrated, your blood volume can actually drop. A reduction in blood volume causes less oxygen to reach muscles, resulting in fatigue and loss of coordination. Your brain's oxygen supply is also reduced, leading to reduced concentration. Allowed to continue, dehydration can cause dizziness and loss of consciousness.

As you work to increase your level of fitness, keep in mind that an effective workout regimen depends largely on your ability to avoid fatigue and stay focused. Keeping well hydrated will allow you to just that.

YOUR FITNESS PROFILE

This chapter includes a series of worksheets that will help you ascertain your current fitness profile. These worksheets will also be used as a baseline so that you can measure your progress. Take the time to fill out each worksheet. Be honest and accurate with your responses. Since you should consult your healthcare provider before starting a new fitness program, you can ask him or her for any information you don't already have at hand.

Your Personal Health Profile Worksheet

MEASUREMENTS	INITIAL	3 MONTHS	6 MONTHS	9 MONTHS	12 MONTHS
Weight					
Body Fat %					
Body Mass Index					
Total Cholesterol					
HDL Cholesterol					
LDL Cholesterol					
Blood Pressure					
Glucose					
Physical Activity mins/day					
Smoking per day					
Alcoholic Drinks per week					

YOUR FITNESS PROFILE

PHYSICAL ACTIVITY READINESS QUESTIONNAIRE

It is important to make sure your body is in proper working order before beginning any fitness routine. Take a moment to go through the following questions. If you answer yes to any of the following questions, please see a medical professional.

Have you ever been told by a medical professional that you have a heart condition?

_____

Do you feel pain in your chest during physical activity?

_____

Have you experienced chest pain in the last month when not engaged in strenuous physical activity?

_____

Have you ever lost consciousness or lost your balance because you became dizzy while engaging in physical activity?

_____

Have you ever lost your balance or lost consciousness when not undergoing physical activity?

_____

Do you suffer from joint or bone ailments or injuries that could be exacerbated by physical activity?

_____

YOUR FITNESS PROFILE

re you taking prescription drugs for high blood pressure or
ny heart condition?

_____

o you know of any other reason why you should not engage
 physical activity?

_____

ITNESS HISTORY

t what age were you in your best physical shape?

_____

ave you ever participated in a workout program? When?

_____

ow long did you stay with the program?

_____

What did the program include?

_____

What lead you to or inspired you to get into shape now?

_____

What will ensure these obstacles do not inhibit you this time?

_____

YOUR FITNESS PROFILE

What obstacles have kept you from meeting your previous fitness goals?

_____

Rate your current fitness level on a scale of 1-10 (1=Worst 10=Best)?

_____

YOUR FITNESS GOALS

By first identifying your goals, you can create a specific workout routine to help you achieve them. Your goals should be specific, quantifiable, realistic and time-based. Fill out the following surveys honestly and with a critical eye. You'll be able to use the resulting information to inspire yourself and ward off possible fitness pitfalls.

FITNESS PREFERENCES

What do you want to accomplish with your workout program?
(Check the boxes next to the goals that are most important to you.)

☐ Improve cardiovascular fitness/endurance

☐ Improve diet and or eating habits

☐ Improve flexibility

☐ Improve health

☐ Improve strength

☐ Improve muscle tone & shape

☐ Increase energy

☐ Gain weight

☐ Lose weight

☐ Prevent injury and/or Rehabilitate injury

☐ Reduce cholesterol

☐ Reduce blood pressure

☐ Reduce risk of disease

☐ Reduce stress

☐ Train for a sports-specific event

☐ Other: _____

☐ Other: _____

YOUR FITNESS GOALS

What types of physical activity do you enjoy and why?

_____

What types of physical activity do you dislike and why?

_____

Do you prefer to exercise alone, with a partner, or in a group?
Why?

_____

WORKOUT PLAN QUESTIONNAIRE

A successful workout plan is one that includes activities yo
enjoy. Be honest in answering the following questions and yo
will be able to develop a plan you can maintain.

Which types of physical activity do you enjoy participating in?

- ☐ Aerobics
- ☐ Active gardening
- ☐ Backpacking
- ☐ Baseball/softball
- ☐ Bicycling/spinning
- ☐ Climbing
- ☐ Cross country skiing
- ☐ Dancing
- ☐ Downhill skiing

- ☐ Football
- ☐ Golfing
- ☐ Hiking
- ☐ Hockey
- ☐ Jogging/running
- ☐ Jump roping
- ☐ Martial arts
- ☐ Pilates
- ☐ Racquetball/handball

YOUR FITNESS GOALS

. . . .

Which types of physical activity do you enjoy
participating in? (Cont.)

☐ Roller blading	☐ Swimming
☐ Rowing	☐ Tennis
☐ Soccer	☐ Volleyball
☐ Skating	☐ Walking
☐ Stair/bench stepping	☐ Weight training
☐ Stretching	☐ Yoga

How many times a week do you want to work out?

- ☐ 1-2 days
- ☐ 2-3 days
- ☐ 3-4 days
- ☐ 5+ days

How long will each session be?

- ☐ 10-20 minutes
- ☐ 20-30 minutes
- ☐ 30-40 minutes
- ☐ 50 + minutes

What days of the week do you have available for exercising?

☐ Mon. ☐ Tues. ☐ Wed. ☐ Thurs. ☐ Fri. ☐ Sat. ☐ Sun.

Notes: _____

YOUR FITNESS GOALS

How will you warm-up and cool down for each workout?

_____

_____

What is your secondary plan if your original workout plan doesn't work?

_____

_____

If exercising outside, do you have a contingency plan for bad weather?

_____

_____

How will you measure your progress?

_____

_____

How long do you think it will take to reach your goal?

_____

_____

YOUR FITNESS GOALS

. . . .

EXERCISE EXCUSES/SOLUTIONS TABLE

EXCUSES	SOLUTIONS
I can't exercise because I'm too tired	I'll workout for 5 minutes & see if I'm still tired
I can't exercise because the gym is too far away	I'll workout at home, maybe go for a walk or do a fitness DVD
I can't exercise because I'm too sore	I'll focus on my stretching, by stretching I will help alleviate soreness and decrease the chances of further injury.
I can't exercise because I'm embarrassed about my body	That's the best reason to workout, not working out will leave your mind time to worry and wallow.
I can't exercise because I'm embarrassed about my body	Play with your kids, playing sports with your children will give an opportunity to bond with them over something they enjoy
I can't exercise because...	
I can't exercise because...	
I can't exercise because...	

NOTES

YOUR WORKOUT SCHEDULE

When creating your workout schedule, consider what you are trying to achieve. Your goals will determine the type of activity, intensity, frequency, and duration of your workouts. If your goal is to lose weight, you will probably want to focus on cardiovascular activities, while those looking to gain weight and build muscle mass will need to focus on weight training. Review your fitness goals questionnaire and pinpoint the main goals. That way you can tailor your program to achieve the maximum results. Take into account your age, current health and fitness level, personal interests, and schedule.

As you develop your workout program, remember that it should include all three components of fitness: cardiovascular conditioning, strength, and flexibility. Training in all three areas will improve your performance in your target area while enhancing your overall fitness. Another important aspect of each workout session is proper warm-up and cool-down activities. Be sure to include both of these in your program.

As you schedule your workouts for each week, be sure to take 1 day to rest. It's just as important to allow your body to recover and rebuild as it is to train hard. If you don't allow proper time for your body to heal and recuperate, you will slow your progress and may never reach your goals.

If you are still unsure of where to begin, below are some activities that you should include in your workout program. You can modify this program gradually as your endurance, strength and skill levels improve.

YOUR WORKOUT SCHEDULE

Warm-up: 5-10 minutes of low intensity/low impact exercise such as walking, slow jogging, knee lifts, arm circles or trunk rotations.

Strength training: Aim for at least two 30-minute sessions per week that may include free weights, weight machines, resistance equipment, muscular endurance training and toning activities such as power yoga or pilates. Be sure to include activities that exercise each of the major muscle groups in these sessions.

Cardiovascular training: Participate in a 30-minute session of aerobic activity at least three times a week. You want to make sure the activity is continuous and is vigorous enough to require increased oxygen consumption. You should breathe hard, but not be so short of breath that you can't carry on a conversation. Typical activities include jogging/running, elliptical training, bicycling/spinning, cardio classes such as step aerobics, kick boxing, and aerobic dance.

Flexibility training: Do 10-15 minutes of stretching per day. An easy way to incorporate flexibility training is by stretching for several minutes after your warm-up and during your cool-down.

Cool-down: Expect to take 5-10 minutes to cool down after your session. Your cool-down can include slow walking or low intensity or low impact exercises with your stretching. Allow your heart rate, breathing and body temperature to gradually drop to normal levels. Use this time to relax and recover from your workout.

YOUR WORKOUT SCHEDULE

· ·

YOUR WORKOUT PROGRAM WORKSHEET

Using what you have learned in this book, fill out the following worksheet to create your personalized workout program.

I. CARDIOVASCULAR TRAINING

Describe your cardiovascular training program:

_____

_____

_____

How many training sessions do you plan per week?

_____

How long will each session last?

_____

II. STRENGTH TRAINING

Describe your strength training program.

_____

_____

_____

_____

_____

YOUR WORKOUT SCHEDULE

How many training sessions do you plan per week?

_____

How long will each session last?

_____

III. FLEXIBILITY TRAINING

Describe your flexibility training program.

_____

_____

_____

_____

_____

How many training sessions do you plan per week?

_____

How long will each session last?

_____

YOUR WORKOUT SCHEDULE

IV. WEEKLY WORKOUT SCHEDULE

Once you have completed the previous sections, fill out the following chart to create a weekly workout schedule.

WEEKLY WORKOUT SCHEDULE			
DAYS OF THE WEEK	CARDIO TRAINING	STRENGTH TRAINING	FLEXIBILITY TRAINING
MONDAY			
TUESDAY			
WEDNESDAY			
THURSDAY			
FRIDAY			
SATURDAY			
SUNDAY			

YOUR WORKOUT SCHEDULE

TRACKING YOUR RESULTS WORKSHEET

Use the following worksheet to keep track of your progress over the next 6 months. Write down your initial measurements.

Initial Measurements:

DATE: / /

Weight		Chest		Thigh	
Body Fat %		Waist		Bicep	
BMI		Hips		Other	

Notes:

_____

_____

_____

_____

_____

_____

_____

_____

_____

YOUR WORKOUT SCHEDULE

Monthly Measurements:

	MONTH 1	MONTH 2	MONTH 3	MONTH 4	MONTH 5	MONTH 6
Weight						
Body Fat %						
BMI						
Chest						
Waist						
Hips						
Thigh						
Bicep						
Other						

YOUR WORKOUT SCHEDULE

PHOTO PROGRESS PAGE

Take an initial photo when you begin your workout program. In one month, take another photo place it below your initial photo. Continue replacing the "current photo" as you see progress on your physical appearance. Be proud of your success!

PLACE INITIAL PHOTO HERE

DATE:
/   /

PLACE CURRENT PHOTO HERE
(Change this picture as you see progress on your physical look.)

DATE:
/   /

USING THE WORKOUT JOURNAL PAGES

To make the most of your workouts, you should keep track of your progress so that you can see yourself approaching your fitness goals. Keeping track of your progress on a daily and weekly basis is the best way to stay motivated and continue working on your fitness program. You can also quickly tell if your progress is slowing down and take action to get yourself back on track. The pages that follow will help you make the most of your fitness program.

GETTING STARTED

Begin with a journal page for Week 1. Take a moment at the start of each day to weigh yourself. For consistency, do this with no clothes and as soon as you wake up in the morning. Record your daily weight in the space provided on each journal page. Read the helpful tip for each day. The daily tip may give you ideas for new exercises or modifications to your routine, or may provide support and motivation.

CARDIOVASCULAR EXERCISE

Each day, make note of any exercise you do to build cardiovascular fitness. Write down how many minutes you spent on the exercise. Depending on the type of exercise, it may also be appropriate to note the distance and pace involved. Pay close attention to your progress. Are cardio workouts getting easier? Do you think it is time to increase the intensity or length

USING THE WORKOUT JOURNAL PAGES

of your workout time? What changes, if any, do you want to make? A great place to note these thoughts are in the End-of-the-Week Wrap-Ups pages.

STRENGTH TRAINING

Use a similar procedure for the strength training section. Note the exercises you do, the amount of weight used, the number of sets, and the number of repetitions for each set.

FLEXIBILITY, RELAXATION, MEDITATION

Make certain that you note the exercises you do to increase flexibility, relaxation, and meditation. Keep track of the time you spend on this very important aspect of fitness training. If there is an exercise that seems particularly helpful or one that you want to concentrate on in the future, it can be beneficial to record these thoughts in the Notes/Reminders section.

WATER INTAKE

Hydration is crucial to the success of your fitness plan. Strive for a total of eight 8-ounce glasses of water per day. Check off a box for each 8-ounce glass that you drink throughout the day. If you drink water on a regular basis throughout the day, you can maintain a constant level of hydration that will optimize your workouts.

USING THE WORKOUT JOURNAL PAGES

VITAMINS & SUPPLEMENTS

This section is a great daily reminder if you are incorporating additional nutrients into your fitness program. If you are restricting your daily caloric intake, it can be a good idea to take vitamins and supplements. If you choose to do so, write it in your journal and be sure to keep track on a daily basis. You can also assess the effectiveness of your supplements over time by comparing your energy levels to the vitamins that you have taken. Also, if you make changes to food that you eat while on your diet, you may want to consider adapting your supplements as well. When in doubt about specific vitamin recommendations, consult with a health care professional.

ENERGY LEVEL

Determine how your body responds to your fitness program. Document your daily overall energy by checking one of the three boxes in this section. See how your energy correlates to the types of exercises you have done for each day. For instance, if you notice that cardiovascular training helps you get through your day with more energy, incorporate a few extra minutes into your workout plan. As you uncover these relationships, make adjustments as needed to help you feel your best.

CALORIES BURNED

This section will allow you to document the calories burned each day. This information can help you recognize behaviors or habits that may lead to a successful fitness journey. It is also a

. . . .

source of reference to help you maintain your ideal body weigh in the future. Refer to the chart on page 40 to determine how many calories you are burning through the activities you do each day.

Weight loss is determined by the amount of calories consumed versus the amount burned. If you happen to have a "bad eating" day, you can try to make up for the excess calories by adding an additional exercise routine the following day. Since you will be recording this number on a daily basis, motivate yourself by incorporating the activities that you enjoy the most.

NOTES/REMINDERS

This section will help you observe obstacles and solutions throughout this workout journey. Record your thoughts and feelings as you gradually achieve your fitness and weight-loss goals. Stay motivated by recording positive results and reflecting on your progress. If for any reason you did not meet your daily goal, reflect on the factors that kept you from your goal and write them down in this section. You can then decide on any changes to your fitness plan that will help you stay on track. Incorporate these improvements into the following day.

END-OF-THE-WEEK WRAP-UP

At the end of each week, use the End-of-the-Week Wrap-Up pages to record your start and end weight, energy level for the week, and total calories burned for the week. Also record how

USING THE WORKOUT JOURNAL PAGES

. . . .

many days you successfully tracked your workouts (although you should aim to do it every day). There is also space to write down how you felt for the week and goals for the following week. Assessing your mood, progress, achievements, and also setbacks will help you prepare for the upcoming week. Don't get bogged down in minor setbacks or obstacles; instead, reward yourself for each small step of success along the way. The End-of-the-Week Wrap-Up pages will give you an accurate picture of your accomplishments for each week and goals for the upcoming week.

MONDAY

CARDIOVASCULAR EXERCISE:

EXERCISE TYPE	TIME/DISTANCE/PACE
Elliptical machine	30mins/3mi/level 5

STRENGTH TRAINING:

EXERCISE TYPE	WEIGHT	SETS	REPS
Squats w/weights	15	3	10
Tricep extensions	10	3	12
Bicep curls	20	2	12
Sit-ups	0		25

EXAMPLE

FLEXIBILITY, MEDITATION:

ACTIVITY PERFORMED	MINUTES
Warm-up stretches	10 mins
Cool-down stretches	10 mins

NOTES/REMINDERS:
Do 15 minutes of meditation before
work tomorrow. Drink 8 glasses of
water!

WEIGHT:
147

WATER INTAKE:
# of 8oz. glasses
☑ ☑ ☑ ☑
☑ ☑ ☐ ☐

**VITAMINS &
SUPPLEMENTS:**
Calcium

ENERGY LEVEL:
☐ low
☑ medium
☐ high

**CALORIES
BURNED:**
500

DATE:

MONDAY

/ /

CARDIOVASCULAR EXERCISE:

EXERCISE TYPE   TIME/DISTANCE/PACE

STRENGTH TRAINING:

EXERCISE TYPE   WEIGHT   SETS   REPS

FLEXIBILITY, RELAXATION MEDITATION:

ACTIVITY PERFORMED   MINUTES

NOTES/REMINDERS:

WEIGHT:

WATER INTAKE:
# of 8oz. glasses
☐ ☐ ☐ ☐
☐ ☐ ☐ ☐

VITAMINS &
SUPPLEMENTS:

ENERGY LEVEL:
☐ low
☐ medium
☐ high

CALORIES
BURNED:

TUESDAY

DATE: __ / __ / __

WEIGHT:

WATER INTAKE:
# of 8oz. glasses
☐ ☐ ☐ ☐
☐ ☐ ☐ ☐

VITAMINS & SUPPLEMENTS:

_____

_____

_____

_____

_____

_____

_____

ENERGY LEVEL:
☐ low
☐ medium
☐ high

CALORIES BURNED:

CARDIOVASCULAR EXERCISE:

EXERCISE TYPE	TIME/DISTANCE/PACE

STRENGTH TRAINING:

EXERCISE TYPE	WEIGHT	SETS	REPS

FLEXIBILITY, RELAXATION MEDITATION:

ACTIVITY PERFORMED	MINUTES

NOTES/REMINDERS:

WEDNESDAY

CARDIOVASCULAR EXERCISE:

EXERCISE TYPE	TIME/DISTANCE/PACE

STRENGTH TRAINING:

EXERCISE TYPE	WEIGHT	SETS	REPS

FLEXIBILITY, RELAXATION MEDITATION:

ACTIVITY PERFORMED	MINUTES

NOTES/REMINDERS:

WEIGHT:

WATER INTAKE:
# of 8oz. glasses
☐ ☐ ☐ ☐
☐ ☐ ☐ ☐

VITAMINS & SUPPLEMENTS:

ENERGY LEVEL:
☐ low
☐ medium
☐ high

CALORIES BURNED:

THURSDAY

DATE: / /

WEIGHT:

WATER INTAKE:
# of 8oz. glasses
☐ ☐ ☐ ☐
☐ ☐ ☐ ☐

VITAMINS & SUPPLEMENTS:

_____

_____

_____

_____

_____

_____

_____

ENERGY LEVEL:
☐ low
☐ medium
☐ high

CALORIES BURNED:

CARDIOVASCULAR EXERCISE:

EXERCISE TYPE	TIME/DISTANCE/PACE

STRENGTH TRAINING:

EXERCISE TYPE	WEIGHT	SETS	REPS

FLEXIBILITY, RELAXATION MEDITATION:

ACTIVITY PERFORMED	MINUTES

NOTES/REMINDERS:

CARDIOVASCULAR EXERCISE:

EXERCISE TYPE	TIME/DISTANCE/PACE

STRENGTH TRAINING:

EXERCISE TYPE	WEIGHT	SETS	REPS

FLEXIBILITY, RELAXATION MEDITATION:

ACTIVITY PERFORMED	MINUTES

NOTES/REMINDERS:

WEIGHT:

WATER INTAKE:
# of 8oz. glasses
☐ ☐ ☐ ☐
☐ ☐ ☐ ☐

VITAMINS &
SUPPLEMENTS:

ENERGY LEVEL:
☐ low
☐ medium
☐ high

CALORIES
BURNED:

SATURDAY

DATE: __ / __ / __

WEIGHT:

WATER INTAKE:
# of 8oz. glasses
☐ ☐ ☐ ☐
☐ ☐ ☐ ☐

VITAMINS & SUPPLEMENTS:

_____
_____
_____
_____
_____
_____
_____

ENERGY LEVEL:
☐ low
☐ medium
☐ high

CALORIES BURNED:

CARDIOVASCULAR EXERCISE:

EXERCISE TYPE	TIME/DISTANCE/PACE

STRENGTH TRAINING:

EXERCISE TYPE	WEIGHT	SETS	REPS

FLEXIBILITY, RELAXATION MEDITATION:

ACTIVITY PERFORMED	MINUTES

NOTES/REMINDERS:

DATE:

/ /

SUNDAY

CARDIOVASCULAR EXERCISE:

EXERCISE TYPE	TIME/DISTANCE/PACE

STRENGTH TRAINING:

EXERCISE TYPE	WEIGHT	SETS	REPS

FLEXIBILITY, RELAXATION MEDITATION:

ACTIVITY PERFORMED	MINUTES

NOTES/REMINDERS:

WEIGHT:

WATER INTAKE:
# of 8oz. glasses
☐ ☐ ☐ ☐
☐ ☐ ☐ ☐

VITAMINS &
SUPPLEMENTS:

ENERGY LEVEL:
☐ low
☐ medium
☐ high

CALORIES
BURNED:

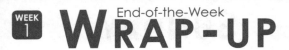

End-of-the-Week
WRAP-UP

| WEEKLY ENERGY LEVEL: | START WEIGHT: | END WEIGHT: | WEEKLY CALORIES BURNED: |

☐ low ☐ med ☐ high

DAYS I WORKED OUT:

☐ Mon. ☐ Tues. ☐ Wed. ☐ Thurs. ☐ Fri. ☐ Sat. ☐ Sun.

HOW I FELT THIS WEEK:

_____

_____

_____

_____

_____

GOALS FOR NEXT WEEK:

_____

_____

_____

_____

_____

NOTES/REMINDERS:

DATE:

__ / __ / __

MONDAY

CARDIOVASCULAR EXERCISE:

EXERCISE TYPE	TIME/DISTANCE/PACE

STRENGTH TRAINING:

EXERCISE TYPE	WEIGHT	SETS	REPS

FLEXIBILITY, RELAXATION MEDITATION:

ACTIVITY PERFORMED	MINUTES

NOTES/REMINDERS:

WEIGHT:

WATER INTAKE:
# of 8oz. glasses
☐ ☐ ☐ ☐
☐ ☐ ☐ ☐

VITAMINS & SUPPLEMENTS:

ENERGY LEVEL:
☐ low
☐ medium
☐ high

CALORIES BURNED:

TUESDAY

DATE: / /

WEIGHT:

WATER INTAKE:
# of 8oz. glasses
☐ ☐ ☐ ☐
☐ ☐ ☐ ☐

VITAMINS & SUPPLEMENTS:

_____
_____
_____
_____
_____
_____
_____

ENERGY LEVEL:
☐ low
☐ medium
☐ high

CALORIES BURNED:

CARDIOVASCULAR EXERCISE:

EXERCISE TYPE	TIME/DISTANCE/PACE

STRENGTH TRAINING:

EXERCISE TYPE	WEIGHT	SETS	REPS

FLEXIBILITY, RELAXATION MEDITATION:

ACTIVITY PERFORMED	MINUTES

NOTES/REMINDERS:

CARDIOVASCULAR EXERCISE:

EXERCISE TYPE	TIME/DISTANCE/PACE

STRENGTH TRAINING:

EXERCISE TYPE	WEIGHT	SETS	REPS

FLEXIBILITY, RELAXATION MEDITATION:

ACTIVITY PERFORMED	MINUTES

NOTES/REMINDERS:

WEIGHT:

WATER INTAKE:
# of 8oz. glasses
☐ ☐ ☐ ☐
☐ ☐ ☐ ☐

**VITAMINS &
SUPPLEMENTS:**

ENERGY LEVEL:
☐ low
☐ medium
☐ high

**CALORIES
BURNED:**

THURSDAY

DATE: / /

WEIGHT:

WATER INTAKE:
# of 8oz. glasses
☐ ☐ ☐ ☐
☐ ☐ ☐ ☐

VITAMINS & SUPPLEMENTS:

_____

_____

_____

_____

_____

_____

_____

ENERGY LEVEL:
☐ low
☐ medium
☐ high

CALORIES BURNED:

CARDIOVASCULAR EXERCISE:

EXERCISE TYPE	TIME/DISTANCE/PACE

STRENGTH TRAINING:

EXERCISE TYPE	WEIGHT	SETS	REPS

FLEXIBILITY, RELAXATION MEDITATION:

ACTIVITY PERFORMED	MINUTES

NOTES/REMINDERS:

DATE:
___/___/___

FRIDAY

CARDIOVASCULAR EXERCISE:

EXERCISE TYPE	TIME/DISTANCE/PACE

STRENGTH TRAINING:

EXERCISE TYPE	WEIGHT	SETS	REPS

FLEXIBILITY, RELAXATION MEDITATION:

ACTIVITY PERFORMED	MINUTES

NOTES/REMINDERS:

WEIGHT:

WATER INTAKE:
# of 8oz. glasses
☐ ☐ ☐ ☐
☐ ☐ ☐ ☐

VITAMINS & SUPPLEMENTS:

ENERGY LEVEL:
☐ low
☐ medium
☐ high

CALORIES BURNED:

SATURDAY

DATE: / /

WEIGHT:

WATER INTAKE:
of 8oz. glasses
☐ ☐ ☐
☐ ☐ ☐

VITAMINS & SUPPLEMENTS:

_____
_____
_____
_____
_____
_____
_____
_____

ENERGY LEVEL:
☐ low
☐ medium
☐ high

CALORIES BURNED:

CARDIOVASCULAR EXERCISE:

EXERCISE TYPE	TIME/DISTANCE/PACE

STRENGTH TRAINING:

EXERCISE TYPE	WEIGHT	SETS	REPS

FLEXIBILITY, RELAXATION MEDITATION:

ACTIVITY PERFORMED	MINUTES

NOTES/REMINDERS:

DATE:
___/___/___

SUNDAY

CARDIOVASCULAR EXERCISE:

EXERCISE TYPE	TIME/DISTANCE/PACE

WEIGHT:

WATER INTAKE:
# of 8oz. glasses
☐ ☐ ☐ ☐
☐ ☐ ☐ ☐

STRENGTH TRAINING:

EXERCISE TYPE	WEIGHT	SETS	REPS

**VITAMINS &
SUPPLEMENTS:**

FLEXIBILITY, RELAXATION MEDITATION:

ACTIVITY PERFORMED	MINUTES

ENERGY LEVEL:
☐ low
☐ medium
☐ high

NOTES/REMINDERS:

**CALORIES
BURNED:**

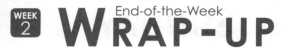

WEEKLY ENERGY LEVEL:

☐ low ☐ med ☐ high

START WEIGHT:

END WEIGHT:

WEEKLY CALORIES BURNED:

DAYS I WORKED OUT:

☐ Mon. ☐ Tues. ☐ Wed. ☐ Thurs. ☐ Fri. ☐ Sat. ☐ Sun.

HOW I FELT THIS WEEK:

_____

_____

_____

_____

GOALS FOR NEXT WEEK:

_____

_____

_____

_____

_____

NOTES/REMINDERS:

DATE:
___/___/___

MONDAY

CARDIOVASCULAR EXERCISE:

EXERCISE TYPE	TIME/DISTANCE/PACE

WEIGHT:

WATER INTAKE:
# of 8oz. glasses
☐ ☐ ☐ ☐
☐ ☐ ☐ ☐

STRENGTH TRAINING:

EXERCISE TYPE	WEIGHT	SETS	REPS

VITAMINS & SUPPLEMENTS:

FLEXIBILITY, RELAXATION MEDITATION:

ACTIVITY PERFORMED	MINUTES

ENERGY LEVEL:
☐ low
☐ medium
☐ high

NOTES/REMINDERS:

CALORIES BURNED:

TUESDAY

DATE: ___ / ___ / ___

WEIGHT:

WATER INTAKE:
# of 8oz. glasses

☐ ☐ ☐ ☐
☐ ☐ ☐ ☐

VITAMINS & SUPPLEMENTS:

_____
_____
_____
_____
_____
_____
_____

ENERGY LEVEL:
☐ low
☐ medium
☐ high

CALORIES BURNED:

CARDIOVASCULAR EXERCISE:

EXERCISE TYPE	TIME/DISTANCE/PACE

STRENGTH TRAINING:

EXERCISE TYPE	WEIGHT	SETS	REPS

FLEXIBILITY, RELAXATION MEDITATION:

ACTIVITY PERFORMED	MINUTES

NOTES/REMINDERS:

WEDNESDAY

CARDIOVASCULAR EXERCISE:

EXERCISE TYPE	TIME/DISTANCE/PACE

STRENGTH TRAINING:

EXERCISE TYPE	WEIGHT	SETS	REPS

FLEXIBILITY, RELAXATION MEDITATION:

ACTIVITY PERFORMED	MINUTES

NOTES/REMINDERS:

WEIGHT:

WATER INTAKE:
# of 8oz. glasses
☐ ☐ ☐ ☐
☐ ☐ ☐ ☐

VITAMINS & SUPPLEMENTS:

ENERGY LEVEL:
☐ low
☐ medium
☐ high

CALORIES BURNED:

THURSDAY

DATE: __ / __ / __

WEIGHT:

WATER INTAKE:
# of 8oz. glasses
☐ ☐ ☐ ☐
☐ ☐ ☐ ☐

**VITAMINS &
SUPPLEMENTS:**

_____
_____
_____
_____
_____
_____

ENERGY LEVEL:
☐ low
☐ medium
☐ high

**CALORIES
BURNED:**

CARDIOVASCULAR EXERCISE:

EXERCISE TYPE	TIME/DISTANCE/PACE

STRENGTH TRAINING:

EXERCISE TYPE	WEIGHT	SETS	REPS

FLEXIBILITY, RELAXATION MEDITATION:

ACTIVITY PERFORMED	MINUTES

NOTES/REMINDERS:

DATE:
/ /

FRIDAY

CARDIOVASCULAR EXERCISE:

EXERCISE TYPE	TIME/DISTANCE/PACE

STRENGTH TRAINING:

EXERCISE TYPE	WEIGHT	SETS	REPS

FLEXIBILITY, RELAXATION MEDITATION:

ACTIVITY PERFORMED	MINUTES

NOTES/REMINDERS:

WEIGHT:

WATER INTAKE:
# of 8oz. glasses
☐ ☐ ☐ ☐
☐ ☐ ☐ ☐

VITAMINS &
SUPPLEMENTS:

ENERGY LEVEL:
☐ low
☐ medium
☐ high

CALORIES
BURNED:

SATURDAY

DATE: __ / __ / __

WEIGHT:

WATER INTAKE:
# of 8oz. glasses
☐ ☐ ☐ ☐
☐ ☐ ☐ ☐

VITAMINS & SUPPLEMENTS:

_____

_____

_____

_____

_____

_____

_____

ENERGY LEVEL:
☐ low
☐ medium
☐ high

CALORIES BURNED:

CARDIOVASCULAR EXERCISE:

EXERCISE TYPE	TIME/DISTANCE/PACE

STRENGTH TRAINING:

EXERCISE TYPE	WEIGHT	SETS	REPS

FLEXIBILITY, RELAXATION MEDITATION:

ACTIVITY PERFORMED	MINUTES

NOTES/REMINDERS:

DATE:

___/___/___

SUNDAY

CARDIOVASCULAR EXERCISE:

EXERCISE TYPE	TIME/DISTANCE/PACE

STRENGTH TRAINING:

EXERCISE TYPE	WEIGHT	SETS	REPS

FLEXIBILITY, RELAXATION MEDITATION:

ACTIVITY PERFORMED	MINUTES

NOTES/REMINDERS:

WEIGHT:

WATER INTAKE:
# of 8oz. glasses
☐ ☐ ☐ ☐
☐ ☐ ☐ ☐

VITAMINS & SUPPLEMENTS:

ENERGY LEVEL:
☐ low
☐ medium
☐ high

CALORIES BURNED:

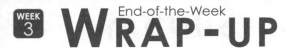

WEEKLY ENERGY LEVEL:

☐ low ☐ med ☐ high

START WEIGHT:

END WEIGHT:

WEEKLY CALORIES BURNED:

DAYS I WORKED OUT:

☐ Mon. ☐ Tues. ☐ Wed. ☐ Thurs. ☐ Fri. ☐ Sat. ☐ Sun.

HOW I FELT THIS WEEK:

_____

_____

_____

_____

GOALS FOR NEXT WEEK:

_____

_____

_____

_____

_____

NOTES/REMINDERS:

DATE:

/ /

MONDAY

CARDIOVASCULAR EXERCISE:

EXERCISE TYPE	TIME/DISTANCE/PACE

WEIGHT:

WATER INTAKE:
# of 8oz. glasses

☐ ☐ ☐ ☐
☐ ☐ ☐ ☐

STRENGTH TRAINING:

EXERCISE TYPE	WEIGHT	SETS	REPS

**VITAMINS &
SUPPLEMENTS:**

FLEXIBILITY, RELAXATION MEDITATION:

ACTIVITY PERFORMED	MINUTES

ENERGY LEVEL:
☐ low
☐ medium
☐ high

NOTES/REMINDERS:

**CALORIES
BURNED:**

TUESDAY

DATE: _ / _ / _

WEIGHT:

WATER INTAKE:
# of 8oz. glasses
☐ ☐ ☐ ☐
☐ ☐ ☐ ☐

VITAMINS & SUPPLEMENTS:

_____

_____

_____

_____

_____

_____

ENERGY LEVEL:
☐ low
☐ medium
☐ high

CALORIES BURNED:

CARDIOVASCULAR EXERCISE:

EXERCISE TYPE	TIME/DISTANCE/PACE

STRENGTH TRAINING:

EXERCISE TYPE	WEIGHT	SETS	REPS

FLEXIBILITY, RELAXATION MEDITATION:

ACTIVITY PERFORMED	MINUTES

NOTES/REMINDERS:

CARDIOVASCULAR EXERCISE:

EXERCISE TYPE	TIME/DISTANCE/PACE

STRENGTH TRAINING:

EXERCISE TYPE	WEIGHT	SETS	REPS

FLEXIBILITY, RELAXATION MEDITATION:

ACTIVITY PERFORMED	MINUTES

NOTES/REMINDERS:

WEIGHT:

WATER INTAKE:
# of 8oz. glasses
☐ ☐ ☐ ☐
☐ ☐ ☐ ☐

VITAMINS & SUPPLEMENTS:

ENERGY LEVEL:
☐ low
☐ medium
☐ high

CALORIES BURNED:

THURSDAY

DATE:
/   /

WEIGHT:

WATER INTAKE:
# of 8oz. glasses
☐ ☐ ☐ ☐
☐ ☐ ☐ ☐

**VITAMINS &
SUPPLEMENTS:**

_____

_____

_____

_____

_____

_____

_____

ENERGY LEVEL:
☐ low
☐ medium
☐ high

**CALORIES
BURNED:**

CARDIOVASCULAR EXERCISE:

EXERCISE TYPE	TIME/DISTANCE/PACE

STRENGTH TRAINING:

EXERCISE TYPE	WEIGHT	SETS	REPS

FLEXIBILITY, RELAXATION MEDITATION:

ACTIVITY PERFORMED	MINUTES

NOTES/REMINDERS:

CARDIOVASCULAR EXERCISE:

EXERCISE TYPE	TIME/DISTANCE/PACE

STRENGTH TRAINING:

EXERCISE TYPE	WEIGHT	SETS	REPS

FLEXIBILITY, RELAXATION MEDITATION:

ACTIVITY PERFORMED	MINUTES

NOTES/REMINDERS:

WEIGHT:

WATER INTAKE:
# of 8oz. glasses
☐ ☐ ☐ ☐
☐ ☐ ☐ ☐

**VITAMINS &
SUPPLEMENTS:**

ENERGY LEVEL:
☐ low
☐ medium
☐ high

**CALORIES
BURNED:**

SATURDAY

DATE: __ / __ / __

WEIGHT:

WATER INTAKE:
# of 8oz. glasses
☐ ☐ ☐ ☐
☐ ☐ ☐ ☐

**VITAMINS &
SUPPLEMENTS:**

ENERGY LEVEL:
☐ low
☐ medium
☐ high

**CALORIES
BURNED:**

CARDIOVASCULAR EXERCISE:

EXERCISE TYPE	TIME/DISTANCE/PACE

STRENGTH TRAINING:

EXERCISE TYPE	WEIGHT	SETS	REPS

FLEXIBILITY, RELAXATION MEDITATION:

ACTIVITY PERFORMED	MINUTES

NOTES/REMINDERS:

DATE:
/ /

SUNDAY

CARDIOVASCULAR EXERCISE:

EXERCISE TYPE	TIME/DISTANCE/PACE

STRENGTH TRAINING:

EXERCISE TYPE	WEIGHT	SETS	REPS

FLEXIBILITY, RELAXATION MEDITATION:

ACTIVITY PERFORMED	MINUTES

NOTES/REMINDERS:

WEIGHT:

WATER INTAKE:
# of 8oz. glasses
☐ ☐ ☐ ☐
☐ ☐ ☐ ☐

VITAMINS & SUPPLEMENTS:

ENERGY LEVEL:
☐ low
☐ medium
☐ high

CALORIES BURNED:

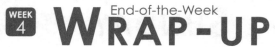

End-of-the-Week
WRAP-UP

WEEKLY ENERGY LEVEL:

☐ low ☐ med ☐ high

START WEIGHT:

END WEIGHT:

WEEKLY CALORIES BURNED:

DAYS I WORKED OUT:

☐ Mon. ☐ Tues. ☐ Wed. ☐ Thurs. ☐ Fri. ☐ Sat. ☐ Sun.

HOW I FELT THIS WEEK:

GOALS FOR NEXT WEEK:

NOTES/REMINDERS:

DATE:

/ /

MONDAY

CARDIOVASCULAR EXERCISE:

EXERCISE TYPE	TIME/DISTANCE/PACE

STRENGTH TRAINING:

EXERCISE TYPE	WEIGHT	SETS	REPS

FLEXIBILITY, RELAXATION MEDITATION:

ACTIVITY PERFORMED	MINUTES

NOTES/REMINDERS:

WEIGHT:

WATER INTAKE:
# of 8oz. glasses
☐ ☐ ☐ ☐
☐ ☐ ☐ ☐

VITAMINS &
SUPPLEMENTS:

ENERGY LEVEL:
☐ low
☐ medium
☐ high

CALORIES
BURNED:

TUESDAY

DATE: / /

WEIGHT:

WATER INTAKE:
# of 8oz. glasses
☐ ☐ ☐ ☐
☐ ☐ ☐ ☐

VITAMINS & SUPPLEMENTS:

ENERGY LEVEL:
☐ low
☐ medium
☐ high

CALORIES BURNED:

CARDIOVASCULAR EXERCISE:

EXERCISE TYPE	TIME/DISTANCE/PACE

STRENGTH TRAINING:

EXERCISE TYPE	WEIGHT	SETS	REPS

FLEXIBILITY, RELAXATION MEDITATION:

ACTIVITY PERFORMED	MINUTES

NOTES/REMINDERS:

WEDNESDAY

CARDIOVASCULAR EXERCISE:

EXERCISE TYPE   **TIME/DISTANCE/PACE**

STRENGTH TRAINING:

EXERCISE TYPE   **WEIGHT SETS REPS**

FLEXIBILITY, RELAXATION MEDITATION:

ACTIVITY PERFORMED   **MINUTES**

NOTES/REMINDERS:

WEIGHT:

WATER INTAKE:
# of 8oz. glasses
☐ ☐ ☐ ☐
☐ ☐ ☐ ☐

VITAMINS & SUPPLEMENTS:

ENERGY LEVEL:
☐ low
☐ medium
☐ high

CALORIES BURNED:

THURSDAY

DATE: __ / __ / __

WEIGHT:

WATER INTAKE:
# of 8oz. glasses
☐ ☐ ☐ ☐
☐ ☐ ☐ ☐

VITAMINS & SUPPLEMENTS:

_____
_____
_____
_____
_____
_____
_____

ENERGY LEVEL:
☐ low
☐ medium
☐ high

CALORIES BURNED:

CARDIOVASCULAR EXERCISE:

EXERCISE TYPE	TIME/DISTANCE/PACE

STRENGTH TRAINING:

EXERCISE TYPE	WEIGHT	SETS	REPS

FLEXIBILITY, RELAXATION MEDITATION:

ACTIVITY PERFORMED	MINUTES

NOTES/REMINDERS:

DATE: __/__/__

FRIDAY

CARDIOVASCULAR EXERCISE:

EXERCISE TYPE	TIME/DISTANCE/PACE

STRENGTH TRAINING:

EXERCISE TYPE	WEIGHT	SETS	REPS

FLEXIBILITY, RELAXATION MEDITATION:

ACTIVITY PERFORMED	MINUTES

NOTES/REMINDERS:

WEIGHT:

WATER INTAKE:
# of 8oz. glasses
☐ ☐ ☐ ☐
☐ ☐ ☐ ☐

VITAMINS & SUPPLEMENTS:

ENERGY LEVEL:
☐ low
☐ medium
☐ high

CALORIES BURNED:

SATURDAY

DATE: __/__/__

WEIGHT:

WATER INTAKE:
# of 8oz. glasses
☐ ☐ ☐ ☐
☐ ☐ ☐ ☐

VITAMINS & SUPPLEMENTS:

ENERGY LEVEL:
☐ low
☐ medium
☐ high

CALORIES BURNED:

CARDIOVASCULAR EXERCISE:

EXERCISE TYPE	TIME/DISTANCE/PACE

STRENGTH TRAINING:

EXERCISE TYPE	WEIGHT	SETS	REPS

FLEXIBILITY, RELAXATION MEDITATION:

ACTIVITY PERFORMED	MINUTES

NOTES/REMINDERS:

DATE:

____/____/____

SUNDAY

CARDIOVASCULAR EXERCISE:

EXERCISE TYPE	TIME/DISTANCE/PACE

WEIGHT:

WATER INTAKE:
# of 8oz. glasses

☐ ☐ ☐ ☐
☐ ☐ ☐ ☐

STRENGTH TRAINING:

EXERCISE TYPE	WEIGHT	SETS	REPS

VITAMINS & SUPPLEMENTS:

_____

_____

_____

_____

_____

_____

FLEXIBILITY, RELAXATION MEDITATION:

ACTIVITY PERFORMED	MINUTES

ENERGY LEVEL:
☐ low
☐ medium
☐ high

NOTES/REMINDERS:

CALORIES BURNED:

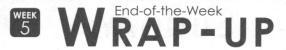

End-of-the-Week
WRAP-UP

WEEKLY ENERGY LEVEL:	START WEIGHT:	END WEIGHT:	WEEKLY CALORIES BURNED:

☐ low ☐ med ☐ high

DAYS I WORKED OUT:
☐ Mon. ☐ Tues. ☐ Wed. ☐ Thurs. ☐ Fri. ☐ Sat. ☐ Sun.

HOW I FELT THIS WEEK:

_____

_____

_____

_____

GOALS FOR NEXT WEEK:

_____

_____

_____

_____

_____

NOTES/REMINDERS:

MONDAY

CARDIOVASCULAR EXERCISE:

EXERCISE TYPE	TIME/DISTANCE/PACE

STRENGTH TRAINING:

EXERCISE TYPE	WEIGHT	SETS	REPS

FLEXIBILITY, RELAXATION MEDITATION:

ACTIVITY PERFORMED	MINUTES

NOTES/REMINDERS:

WEIGHT:

WATER INTAKE:
# of 8oz. glasses
☐ ☐ ☐ ☐
☐ ☐ ☐ ☐

VITAMINS & SUPPLEMENTS:

ENERGY LEVEL:
☐ low
☐ medium
☐ high

CALORIES BURNED:

TUESDAY

DATE: ___/___/___

WEIGHT:

WATER INTAKE:
# of 8oz. glasses
☐ ☐ ☐ ☐
☐ ☐ ☐ ☐

VITAMINS & SUPPLEMENTS:

_____
_____
_____
_____
_____
_____
_____

ENERGY LEVEL:
☐ low
☐ medium
☐ high

CALORIES BURNED:

CARDIOVASCULAR EXERCISE:

EXERCISE TYPE	TIME/DISTANCE/PACE

STRENGTH TRAINING:

EXERCISE TYPE	WEIGHT	SETS	REPS

FLEXIBILITY, RELAXATION MEDITATION:

ACTIVITY PERFORMED	MINUTES

NOTES/REMINDERS:

WEDNESDAY

DATE: __/__/__

CARDIOVASCULAR EXERCISE:

EXERCISE TYPE	TIME/DISTANCE/PACE

STRENGTH TRAINING:

EXERCISE TYPE	WEIGHT	SETS	REPS

FLEXIBILITY, RELAXATION MEDITATION:

ACTIVITY PERFORMED	MINUTES

NOTES/REMINDERS:

WEIGHT:

WATER INTAKE:
# of 8oz. glasses
☐ ☐ ☐ ☐
☐ ☐ ☐ ☐

VITAMINS & SUPPLEMENTS:

ENERGY LEVEL:
☐ low
☐ medium
☐ high

CALORIES BURNED:

THURSDAY

DATE:
/ /

WEIGHT:

WATER INTAKE:
# of 8oz. glasses
☐ ☐ ☐ ☐
☐ ☐ ☐ ☐

VITAMINS & SUPPLEMENTS:

_____

_____

_____

_____

_____

_____

_____

ENERGY LEVEL:
☐ low
☐ medium
☐ high

CALORIES BURNED:

CARDIOVASCULAR EXERCISE:

EXERCISE TYPE	TIME/DISTANCE/PACE

STRENGTH TRAINING:

EXERCISE TYPE	WEIGHT	SETS	REPS

FLEXIBILITY, RELAXATION MEDITATION:

ACTIVITY PERFORMED	MINUTES

NOTES/REMINDERS:

FRIDAY

CARDIOVASCULAR EXERCISE:

EXERCISE TYPE	TIME/DISTANCE/PACE

STRENGTH TRAINING:

EXERCISE TYPE	WEIGHT	SETS	REPS

FLEXIBILITY, RELAXATION MEDITATION:

ACTIVITY PERFORMED	MINUTES

NOTES/REMINDERS:

WEIGHT:

WATER INTAKE:
# of 8oz. glasses
☐ ☐ ☐ ☐
☐ ☐ ☐ ☐

VITAMINS & SUPPLEMENTS:

ENERGY LEVEL:
☐ low
☐ medium
☐ high

CALORIES BURNED:

SATURDAY

DATE: / /

WEIGHT:

WATER INTAKE:
# of 8oz. glasses
☐ ☐ ☐
☐ ☐ ☐

VITAMINS & SUPPLEMENTS:

_____
_____
_____
_____
_____
_____
_____

ENERGY LEVEL:
☐ low
☐ medium
☐ high

CALORIES BURNED:

CARDIOVASCULAR EXERCISE:

EXERCISE TYPE	TIME/DISTANCE/PACE

STRENGTH TRAINING:

EXERCISE TYPE	WEIGHT	SETS	REPS

FLEXIBILITY, RELAXATION MEDITATION:

ACTIVITY PERFORMED	MINUTES

NOTES/REMINDERS:

DATE: / /

SUNDAY

CARDIOVASCULAR EXERCISE:

EXERCISE TYPE	TIME/DISTANCE/PACE

STRENGTH TRAINING:

EXERCISE TYPE	WEIGHT	SETS	REPS

FLEXIBILITY, RELAXATION MEDITATION:

ACTIVITY PERFORMED	MINUTES

NOTES/REMINDERS:

WEIGHT:

WATER INTAKE:
# of 8oz. glasses
☐ ☐ ☐ ☐
☐ ☐ ☐ ☐

VITAMINS & SUPPLEMENTS:

ENERGY LEVEL:
☐ low
☐ medium
☐ high

CALORIES BURNED:

WEEKLY ENERGY LEVEL:	START WEIGHT:	END WEIGHT:	WEEKLY CALORIES BURNED:
☐ low ☐ med ☐ high			

DAYS I WORKED OUT:

☐ Mon. ☐ Tues. ☐ Wed. ☐ Thurs. ☐ Fri. ☐ Sat. ☐ Sun.

HOW I FELT THIS WEEK:

_____

_____

_____

_____

GOALS FOR NEXT WEEK:

_____

_____

_____

_____

_____

NOTES/REMINDERS:

DATE:

___/___/___

MONDAY

CARDIOVASCULAR EXERCISE:

EXERCISE TYPE	TIME/DISTANCE/PACE

STRENGTH TRAINING:

EXERCISE TYPE	WEIGHT	SETS	REPS

FLEXIBILITY, RELAXATION MEDITATION:

ACTIVITY PERFORMED	MINUTES

NOTES/REMINDERS:

WEIGHT:

WATER INTAKE:
# of 8oz. glasses
☐ ☐ ☐ ☐
☐ ☐ ☐ ☐

VITAMINS & SUPPLEMENTS:

ENERGY LEVEL:
☐ low
☐ medium
☐ high

CALORIES BURNED:

TUESDAY

DATE: / /

WEIGHT:

WATER INTAKE:
# of 8oz. glasses
☐ ☐ ☐ ☐
☐ ☐ ☐ ☐

VITAMINS & SUPPLEMENTS:

_____

_____

_____

_____

_____

_____

_____

ENERGY LEVEL:
☐ low
☐ medium
☐ high

CALORIES BURNED:

CARDIOVASCULAR EXERCISE:

EXERCISE TYPE	TIME/DISTANCE/PACE

STRENGTH TRAINING:

EXERCISE TYPE	WEIGHT	SETS	REPS

FLEXIBILITY, RELAXATION MEDITATION:

ACTIVITY PERFORMED	MINUTES

NOTES/REMINDERS:

DATE:
___/___/___

WEDNESDAY

CARDIOVASCULAR EXERCISE:

EXERCISE TYPE	**TIME/DISTANCE/PACE**

STRENGTH TRAINING:

EXERCISE TYPE	**WEIGHT**	**SETS**	**REPS**

FLEXIBILITY, RELAXATION MEDITATION:

ACTIVITY PERFORMED	**MINUTES**

NOTES/REMINDERS:

WEIGHT:

WATER INTAKE:
# of 8oz. glasses
☐ ☐ ☐ ☐
☐ ☐ ☐ ☐

VITAMINS & SUPPLEMENTS:

ENERGY LEVEL:
☐ low
☐ medium
☐ high

CALORIES BURNED:

THURSDAY

DATE: ___ / ___ / ___

WEIGHT:

WATER INTAKE:
# of 8oz. glasses
☐ ☐ ☐
☐ ☐ ☐

VITAMINS & SUPPLEMENTS:

_____
_____
_____
_____
_____
_____
_____

ENERGY LEVEL:
☐ low
☐ medium
☐ high

CALORIES BURNED:

CARDIOVASCULAR EXERCISE:

EXERCISE TYPE	TIME/DISTANCE/PACE

STRENGTH TRAINING:

EXERCISE TYPE	WEIGHT	SETS	REPS

FLEXIBILITY, RELAXATION MEDITATION:

ACTIVITY PERFORMED	MINUTES

NOTES/REMINDERS:

DATE:

/ /

FRIDAY

CARDIOVASCULAR EXERCISE:

EXERCISE TYPE   TIME/DISTANCE/PACE

_____   _____

_____   _____

_____   _____

STRENGTH TRAINING:

EXERCISE TYPE   WEIGHT   SETS   REPS

_____

_____

_____

_____

_____

_____

_____

FLEXIBILITY, RELAXATION MEDITATION:

ACTIVITY PERFORMED   MINUTES

_____   _____

_____   _____

_____   _____

NOTES/REMINDERS:

WEIGHT:

WATER INTAKE:
# of 8oz. glasses
☐ ☐ ☐ ☐
☐ ☐ ☐ ☐

**VITAMINS &
SUPPLEMENTS:**

_____

_____

_____

_____

_____

_____

_____

ENERGY LEVEL:
☐ low
☐ medium
☐ high

**CALORIES
BURNED:**

SATURDAY

DATE: __ / __ / __

WEIGHT:

WATER INTAKE:
# of 8oz. glasses
☐ ☐ ☐ ☐
☐ ☐ ☐ ☐

VITAMINS &
SUPPLEMENTS:
_____
_____
_____
_____
_____
_____
_____
_____

ENERGY LEVEL:
☐ low
☐ medium
☐ high

CALORIES
BURNED:

CARDIOVASCULAR EXERCISE:

EXERCISE TYPE	TIME/DISTANCE/PACE

STRENGTH TRAINING:

EXERCISE TYPE	WEIGHT	SETS	REPS

FLEXIBILITY, RELAXATION MEDITATION:

ACTIVITY PERFORMED	MINUTES

NOTES/REMINDERS:

DATE: __/__/__

SUNDAY

CARDIOVASCULAR EXERCISE:

EXERCISE TYPE	TIME/DISTANCE/PACE

STRENGTH TRAINING:

EXERCISE TYPE	WEIGHT	SETS	REPS

FLEXIBILITY, RELAXATION MEDITATION:

ACTIVITY PERFORMED	MINUTES

NOTES/REMINDERS:

WEIGHT:

WATER INTAKE:
# of 8oz. glasses
☐ ☐ ☐ ☐
☐ ☐ ☐ ☐

VITAMINS & SUPPLEMENTS:

ENERGY LEVEL:
☐ low
☐ medium
☐ high

CALORIES BURNED:

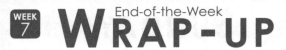

WEEK 7

End-of-the-Week WRAP-UP

WEEKLY ENERGY LEVEL:	START WEIGHT:	END WEIGHT:	WEEKLY CALORIES BURNED:

☐ low ☐ med ☐ high

DAYS I WORKED OUT:

☐ Mon. ☐ Tues. ☐ Wed. ☐ Thurs. ☐ Fri. ☐ Sat. ☐ Sun.

HOW I FELT THIS WEEK:

_____

_____

_____

_____

_____

GOALS FOR NEXT WEEK:

_____

_____

_____

_____

_____

NOTES/REMINDERS:

DATE:

_/_ /_

MONDAY

CARDIOVASCULAR EXERCISE:

EXERCISE TYPE   TIME/DISTANCE/PACE

_____   _____

_____   _____

_____   _____

STRENGTH TRAINING:

EXERCISE TYPE   WEIGHT   SETS   REPS

WEIGHT:

WATER INTAKE:
# of 8oz. glasses
☐ ☐ ☐ ☐
☐ ☐ ☐ ☐

VITAMINS &
SUPPLEMENTS:

_____

_____

_____

_____

_____

FLEXIBILITY, RELAXATION MEDITATION:

ACTIVITY PERFORMED   MINUTES

_____   _____

_____   _____

_____   _____

NOTES/REMINDERS:

ENERGY LEVEL:
☐ low
☐ medium
☐ high

CALORIES
BURNED:

TUESDAY

DATE: / /

WEIGHT:

WATER INTAKE:
# of 8oz. glasses
☐ ☐ ☐ ☐
☐ ☐ ☐ ☐

VITAMINS & SUPPLEMENTS:

_____

_____

_____

_____

_____

_____

_____

ENERGY LEVEL:
☐ low
☐ medium
☐ high

CALORIES BURNED:

CARDIOVASCULAR EXERCISE:

EXERCISE TYPE	TIME/DISTANCE/PACE

STRENGTH TRAINING:

EXERCISE TYPE	WEIGHT	SETS	REPS

FLEXIBILITY, RELAXATION MEDITATION:

ACTIVITY PERFORMED	MINUTES

NOTES/REMINDERS:

WEDNESDAY

CARDIOVASCULAR EXERCISE:

EXERCISE TYPE	TIME/DISTANCE/PACE

STRENGTH TRAINING:

EXERCISE TYPE	WEIGHT	SETS	REPS

FLEXIBILITY, RELAXATION MEDITATION:

ACTIVITY PERFORMED	MINUTES

NOTES/REMINDERS:

WEIGHT:

WATER INTAKE:
# of 8oz. glasses
☐ ☐ ☐ ☐
☐ ☐ ☐ ☐

VITAMINS & SUPPLEMENTS:

ENERGY LEVEL:
☐ low
☐ medium
☐ high

CALORIES BURNED:

THURSDAY

DATE:
/ /

WEIGHT:

WATER INTAKE:
# of 8oz. glasses
☐ ☐ ☐ ☐
☐ ☐ ☐ ☐

**VITAMINS &
SUPPLEMENTS:**

ENERGY LEVEL:
☐ low
☐ medium
☐ high

**CALORIES
BURNED:**

CARDIOVASCULAR EXERCISE:

EXERCISE TYPE	TIME/DISTANCE/PACE

STRENGTH TRAINING:

EXERCISE TYPE	WEIGHT	SETS	REPS

FLEXIBILITY, RELAXATION MEDITATION:

ACTIVITY PERFORMED	MINUTES

NOTES/REMINDERS:

DATE:
/ /

FRIDAY

CARDIOVASCULAR EXERCISE:

EXERCISE TYPE   TIME/DISTANCE/PACE

_____   _____

_____   _____

_____   _____

STRENGTH TRAINING:

EXERCISE TYPE   WEIGHT   SETS   REPS

_____

_____

_____

_____

_____

_____

FLEXIBILITY, RELAXATION MEDITATION:

ACTIVITY PERFORMED   MINUTES

_____   _____

_____   _____

_____   _____

NOTES/REMINDERS:

WEIGHT:

WATER INTAKE:
# of 8oz. glasses
☐ ☐ ☐ ☐
☐ ☐ ☐ ☐

**VITAMINS &
SUPPLEMENTS:**

_____

_____

_____

_____

_____

_____

ENERGY LEVEL:
☐ low
☐ medium
☐ high

**CALORIES
BURNED:**

SATURDAY

DATE: __/__/__

WEIGHT:

WATER INTAKE:
# of 8oz. glasses
☐ ☐ ☐ ☐
☐ ☐ ☐ ☐

**VITAMINS &
SUPPLEMENTS:**

_____
_____
_____
_____
_____
_____
_____
_____

ENERGY LEVEL:
☐ low
☐ medium
☐ high

**CALORIES
BURNED:**

CARDIOVASCULAR EXERCISE:

EXERCISE TYPE	TIME/DISTANCE/PACE

STRENGTH TRAINING:

EXERCISE TYPE	WEIGHT	SETS	REPS

FLEXIBILITY, RELAXATION MEDITATION:

ACTIVITY PERFORMED	MINUTES

NOTES/REMINDERS:

DATE: / /

SUNDAY

CARDIOVASCULAR EXERCISE:

EXERCISE TYPE	TIME/DISTANCE/PACE

STRENGTH TRAINING:

EXERCISE TYPE	WEIGHT	SETS	REPS

FLEXIBILITY, RELAXATION MEDITATION:

ACTIVITY PERFORMED	MINUTES

NOTES/REMINDERS:

WEIGHT:

WATER INTAKE:
# of 8oz. glasses
☐ ☐ ☐ ☐
☐ ☐ ☐ ☐

VITAMINS & SUPPLEMENTS:

ENERGY LEVEL:
☐ low
☐ medium
☐ high

CALORIES BURNED:

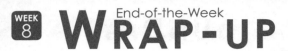

WEEKLY ENERGY LEVEL:

☐ low ☐ med ☐ high

START WEIGHT:

END WEIGHT:

WEEKLY CALORIES BURNED:

DAYS I WORKED OUT:

☐ Mon. ☐ Tues. ☐ Wed. ☐ Thurs. ☐ Fri. ☐ Sat. ☐ Sun.

HOW I FELT THIS WEEK:

_____

_____

_____

_____

_____

GOALS FOR NEXT WEEK:

_____

_____

_____

_____

_____

NOTES/REMINDERS:

DATE:

/ /

MONDAY

CARDIOVASCULAR EXERCISE:

EXERCISE TYPE	TIME/DISTANCE/PACE

STRENGTH TRAINING:

EXERCISE TYPE	WEIGHT	SETS	REPS

FLEXIBILITY, RELAXATION MEDITATION:

ACTIVITY PERFORMED	MINUTES

NOTES/REMINDERS:

WEIGHT:

WATER INTAKE:
# of 8oz. glasses
☐ ☐ ☐ ☐
☐ ☐ ☐ ☐

VITAMINS & SUPPLEMENTS:

ENERGY LEVEL:
☐ low
☐ medium
☐ high

CALORIES BURNED:

TUESDAY

DATE:
/ /

WEIGHT:

WATER INTAKE:
# of 8oz. glasses
☐ ☐ ☐ ☐
☐ ☐ ☐ ☐

**VITAMINS &
SUPPLEMENTS:**

_____

_____

_____

_____

_____

_____

_____

ENERGY LEVEL:
☐ low
☐ medium
☐ high

**CALORIES
BURNED:**

CARDIOVASCULAR EXERCISE:

EXERCISE TYPE	TIME/DISTANCE/PACE

STRENGTH TRAINING:

EXERCISE TYPE	WEIGHT	SETS	REPS

FLEXIBILITY, RELAXATION MEDITATION:

ACTIVITY PERFORMED	MINUTES

NOTES/REMINDERS:

DATE:

___/___/___

WEDNESDAY

CARDIOVASCULAR EXERCISE:

EXERCISE TYPE

TIME/DISTANCE/PACE

STRENGTH TRAINING:

EXERCISE TYPE

WEIGHT **SETS** **REPS**

FLEXIBILITY, RELAXATION MEDITATION:

ACTIVITY PERFORMED

MINUTES

NOTES/REMINDERS:

WEIGHT:

WATER INTAKE:
# of 8oz. glasses

☐ ☐ ☐ ☐
☐ ☐ ☐ ☐

VITAMINS & SUPPLEMENTS:

ENERGY LEVEL:
☐ low
☐ medium
☐ high

CALORIES BURNED:

THURSDAY

DATE: / /

WEIGHT:

WATER INTAKE:
# of 8oz. glasses
☐ ☐ ☐ ☐
☐ ☐ ☐ ☐

VITAMINS & SUPPLEMENTS:

ENERGY LEVEL:
☐ low
☐ medium
☐ high

CALORIES BURNED:

CARDIOVASCULAR EXERCISE:

EXERCISE TYPE	TIME/DISTANCE/PACE

STRENGTH TRAINING:

EXERCISE TYPE	WEIGHT	SETS	REPS

FLEXIBILITY, RELAXATION MEDITATION:

ACTIVITY PERFORMED	MINUTES

NOTES/REMINDERS:

DATE: / /

FRIDAY

CARDIOVASCULAR EXERCISE:

EXERCISE TYPE	TIME/DISTANCE/PACE

WEIGHT:

WATER INTAKE:
# of 8oz. glasses
☐ ☐ ☐ ☐
☐ ☐ ☐ ☐

STRENGTH TRAINING:

EXERCISE TYPE	WEIGHT	SETS	REPS

VITAMINS & SUPPLEMENTS:

FLEXIBILITY, RELAXATION MEDITATION:

ACTIVITY PERFORMED	MINUTES

ENERGY LEVEL:
☐ low
☐ medium
☐ high

NOTES/REMINDERS:

CALORIES BURNED:

SATURDAY

DATE: / /

WEIGHT:

WATER INTAKE:
# of 8oz. glasses
☐ ☐ ☐ ☐
☐ ☐ ☐ ☐

VITAMINS & SUPPLEMENTS:

ENERGY LEVEL:
☐ low
☐ medium
☐ high

CALORIES BURNED:

CARDIOVASCULAR EXERCISE:

EXERCISE TYPE	TIME/DISTANCE/PACE

STRENGTH TRAINING:

EXERCISE TYPE	WEIGHT	SETS	REPS

FLEXIBILITY, RELAXATION MEDITATION:

ACTIVITY PERFORMED	MINUTES

NOTES/REMINDERS:

DATE:

/ /

SUNDAY

CARDIOVASCULAR EXERCISE:

EXERCISE TYPE	TIME/DISTANCE/PACE

WEIGHT:

WATER INTAKE:
# of 8oz. glasses

☐ ☐ ☐ ☐
☐ ☐ ☐ ☐

STRENGTH TRAINING:

EXERCISE TYPE	WEIGHT	SETS	REPS

VITAMINS & SUPPLEMENTS:

_____

_____

_____

_____

_____

_____

_____

FLEXIBILITY, RELAXATION MEDITATION:

ACTIVITY PERFORMED	MINUTES

ENERGY LEVEL:
☐ low
☐ medium
☐ high

NOTES/REMINDERS:

CALORIES BURNED:

End-of-the-Week WRAP-UP

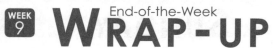

| WEEKLY ENERGY LEVEL: | START WEIGHT: | END WEIGHT: | WEEKLY CALORIES BURNED: |

☐ low ☐ med ☐ high

DAYS I WORKED OUT:
☐ Mon. ☐ Tues. ☐ Wed. ☐ Thurs. ☐ Fri. ☐ Sat. ☐ Sun.

HOW I FELT THIS WEEK:

_____

_____

_____

_____

_____

GOALS FOR NEXT WEEK:

_____

_____

_____

_____

_____

NOTES/REMINDERS:

DATE:
/ /

MONDAY

CARDIOVASCULAR EXERCISE:

EXERCISE TYPE	TIME/DISTANCE/PACE

STRENGTH TRAINING:

EXERCISE TYPE	WEIGHT	SETS	REPS

FLEXIBILITY, RELAXATION MEDITATION:

ACTIVITY PERFORMED	MINUTES

NOTES/REMINDERS:

WEIGHT:

WATER INTAKE:
# of 8oz. glasses
☐ ☐ ☐ ☐
☐ ☐ ☐ ☐

VITAMINS & SUPPLEMENTS:

ENERGY LEVEL:
☐ low
☐ medium
☐ high

CALORIES BURNED:

TUESDAY

DATE:
/ /

WEIGHT:

WATER INTAKE:
# of 8oz. glasses
☐ ☐ ☐ ☐
☐ ☐ ☐ ☐

VITAMINS & SUPPLEMENTS:

_____
_____
_____
_____
_____
_____
_____
_____

ENERGY LEVEL:
☐ low
☐ medium
☐ high

CALORIES BURNED:

CARDIOVASCULAR EXERCISE:

EXERCISE TYPE	TIME/DISTANCE/PACE

STRENGTH TRAINING:

EXERCISE TYPE	WEIGHT	SETS	REPS

FLEXIBILITY, RELAXATION MEDITATION:

ACTIVITY PERFORMED	MINUTES

NOTES/REMINDERS:

CARDIOVASCULAR EXERCISE:

EXERCISE TYPE	TIME/DISTANCE/PACE

STRENGTH TRAINING:

EXERCISE TYPE	WEIGHT	SETS	REPS

FLEXIBILITY, RELAXATION MEDITATION:

ACTIVITY PERFORMED	MINUTES

NOTES/REMINDERS:

WEIGHT:

WATER INTAKE:
# of 8oz. glasses
☐ ☐ ☐ ☐
☐ ☐ ☐ ☐

VITAMINS & SUPPLEMENTS:

ENERGY LEVEL:
☐ low
☐ medium
☐ high

CALORIES BURNED:

THURSDAY

DATE:
/ /

WEIGHT:

WATER INTAKE:
# of 8oz. glasses
☐ ☐ ☐ ☐
☐ ☐ ☐ ☐

**VITAMINS &
SUPPLEMENTS:**

_____

_____

_____

_____

_____

_____

_____

_____

ENERGY LEVEL:
☐ low
☐ medium
☐ high

**CALORIES
BURNED:**

CARDIOVASCULAR EXERCISE:

EXERCISE TYPE	TIME/DISTANCE/PACE

STRENGTH TRAINING:

EXERCISE TYPE	WEIGHT	SETS	REPS

FLEXIBILITY, RELAXATION MEDITATION:

ACTIVITY PERFORMED	MINUTES

NOTES/REMINDERS:

DATE:
/ /

FRIDAY

CARDIOVASCULAR EXERCISE:

EXERCISE TYPE	TIME/DISTANCE/PACE

STRENGTH TRAINING:

EXERCISE TYPE	WEIGHT	SETS	REPS

FLEXIBILITY, RELAXATION MEDITATION:

ACTIVITY PERFORMED	MINUTES

NOTES/REMINDERS:

WEIGHT:

WATER INTAKE:
# of 8oz. glasses
☐ ☐ ☐ ☐
☐ ☐ ☐ ☐

VITAMINS &
SUPPLEMENTS:

ENERGY LEVEL:
☐ low
☐ medium
☐ high

CALORIES
BURNED:

SATURDAY

DATE: / /

WEIGHT:

WATER INTAKE:
# of 8oz. glasses
☐ ☐ ☐ ☐
☐ ☐ ☐ ☐

VITAMINS & SUPPLEMENTS:

_____

_____

_____

_____

_____

_____

_____

ENERGY LEVEL:
☐ low
☐ medium
☐ high

CALORIES BURNED:

CARDIOVASCULAR EXERCISE:

EXERCISE TYPE	TIME/DISTANCE/PACE

STRENGTH TRAINING:

EXERCISE TYPE	WEIGHT	SETS	REPS

FLEXIBILITY, RELAXATION MEDITATION:

ACTIVITY PERFORMED	MINUTES

NOTES/REMINDERS:

DATE:

SUNDAY

/ /

CARDIOVASCULAR EXERCISE:

EXERCISE TYPE	TIME/DISTANCE/PACE

STRENGTH TRAINING:

EXERCISE TYPE	WEIGHT	SETS	REPS

FLEXIBILITY, RELAXATION MEDITATION:

ACTIVITY PERFORMED	MINUTES

NOTES/REMINDERS:

WEIGHT:

WATER INTAKE:
# of 8oz. glasses
☐ ☐ ☐ ☐
☐ ☐ ☐ ☐

VITAMINS &
SUPPLEMENTS:

ENERGY LEVEL:
☐ low
☐ medium
☐ high

CALORIES
BURNED:

End-of-the-Week WRAP-UP

WEEKLY ENERGY LEVEL:	START WEIGHT:	END WEIGHT:	WEEKLY CALORIES BURNED:

☐ low ☐ med ☐ high

DAYS I WORKED OUT:

☐ Mon. ☐ Tues. ☐ Wed. ☐ Thurs. ☐ Fri. ☐ Sat. ☐ Sun.

HOW I FELT THIS WEEK:

_____

_____

_____

_____

_____

GOALS FOR NEXT WEEK:

_____

_____

_____

_____

_____

NOTES/REMINDERS:

DATE:
_/_/_

MONDAY

CARDIOVASCULAR EXERCISE:

EXERCISE TYPE   TIME/DISTANCE/PACE

_____ _____

_____ _____

_____ _____

STRENGTH TRAINING:

EXERCISE TYPE   WEIGHT   SETS   REPS

_____

_____

_____

_____

_____

_____

_____

FLEXIBILITY, RELAXATION MEDITATION:

ACTIVITY PERFORMED   MINUTES

_____ _____

_____ _____

_____ _____

NOTES/REMINDERS:

WEIGHT:

WATER INTAKE:
# of 8oz. glasses
☐ ☐ ☐ ☐
☐ ☐ ☐ ☐

VITAMINS &
SUPPLEMENTS:

_____

_____

_____

_____

_____

_____

_____

ENERGY LEVEL:
☐ low
☐ medium
☐ high

CALORIES
BURNED:

TUESDAY

DATE:
/ /

WEIGHT:

WATER INTAKE:
# of 8oz. glasses
☐ ☐ ☐ ☐
☐ ☐ ☐ ☐

VITAMINS &
SUPPLEMENTS:

_____

_____

_____

_____

_____

_____

_____

ENERGY LEVEL:
☐ low
☐ medium
☐ high

CALORIES
BURNED:

CARDIOVASCULAR EXERCISE:

EXERCISE TYPE	TIME/DISTANCE/PACE

STRENGTH TRAINING:

EXERCISE TYPE	WEIGHT	SETS	REPS

FLEXIBILITY, RELAXATION MEDITATION:

ACTIVITY PERFORMED	MINUTES

NOTES/REMINDERS:

DATE: __/__/__

WEDNESDAY

CARDIOVASCULAR EXERCISE:

EXERCISE TYPE	TIME/DISTANCE/PACE

STRENGTH TRAINING:

EXERCISE TYPE	WEIGHT	SETS	REPS

FLEXIBILITY, RELAXATION MEDITATION:

ACTIVITY PERFORMED	MINUTES

NOTES/REMINDERS:

WEIGHT:

WATER INTAKE:
# of 8oz. glasses
☐ ☐ ☐ ☐
☐ ☐ ☐ ☐

VITAMINS & SUPPLEMENTS:

ENERGY LEVEL:
☐ low
☐ medium
☐ high

CALORIES BURNED:

THURSDAY

DATE:
/ /

WEIGHT:

WATER INTAKE:
# of 8oz. glasses
☐ ☐ ☐ ☐
☐ ☐ ☐ ☐

VITAMINS & SUPPLEMENTS:

ENERGY LEVEL:
☐ low
☐ medium
☐ high

CALORIES BURNED:

CARDIOVASCULAR EXERCISE:

EXERCISE TYPE	TIME/DISTANCE/PACE

STRENGTH TRAINING:

EXERCISE TYPE	WEIGHT	SETS	REPS

FLEXIBILITY, RELAXATION MEDITATION:

ACTIVITY PERFORMED	MINUTES

NOTES/REMINDERS:

DATE:
/ /

FRIDAY

CARDIOVASCULAR EXERCISE:

EXERCISE TYPE	TIME/DISTANCE/PACE

STRENGTH TRAINING:

EXERCISE TYPE	WEIGHT	SETS	REPS

FLEXIBILITY, RELAXATION MEDITATION:

ACTIVITY PERFORMED	MINUTES

NOTES/REMINDERS:

WEIGHT:

WATER INTAKE:
# of 8oz. glasses
☐ ☐ ☐ ☐
☐ ☐ ☐ ☐

VITAMINS & SUPPLEMENTS:

ENERGY LEVEL:
☐ low
☐ medium
☐ high

CALORIES BURNED:

SATURDAY

DATE: / /

WEIGHT:

WATER INTAKE:
# of 8oz. glasses
☐ ☐ ☐ ☐
☐ ☐ ☐ ☐

VITAMINS & SUPPLEMENTS:

_____
_____
_____
_____
_____
_____
_____
_____

ENERGY LEVEL:
☐ low
☐ medium
☐ high

CALORIES BURNED:

CARDIOVASCULAR EXERCISE:

EXERCISE TYPE	TIME/DISTANCE/PACE

STRENGTH TRAINING:

EXERCISE TYPE	WEIGHT	SETS	REPS

FLEXIBILITY, RELAXATION MEDITATION:

ACTIVITY PERFORMED	MINUTES

NOTES/REMINDERS:

DATE:

/ /

SUNDAY

CARDIOVASCULAR EXERCISE:

EXERCISE TYPE	TIME/DISTANCE/PACE

STRENGTH TRAINING:

EXERCISE TYPE	WEIGHT	SETS	REPS

FLEXIBILITY, RELAXATION MEDITATION:

ACTIVITY PERFORMED	MINUTES

NOTES/REMINDERS:

WEIGHT:

WATER INTAKE:
# of 8oz. glasses
☐ ☐ ☐ ☐
☐ ☐ ☐ ☐

VITAMINS & SUPPLEMENTS:

ENERGY LEVEL:
☐ low
☐ medium
☐ high

CALORIES BURNED:

End-of-the-Week WRAP-UP

WEEKLY ENERGY LEVEL: **START WEIGHT:** **END WEIGHT:** **WEEKLY CALORIE BURNED:**

☐ low ☐ med ☐ high

DAYS I WORKED OUT:

☐ Mon. ☐ Tues. ☐ Wed. ☐ Thurs. ☐ Fri. ☐ Sat. ☐ Sun.

HOW I FELT THIS WEEK:

_____

_____

_____

_____

_____

GOALS FOR NEXT WEEK:

_____

_____

_____

_____

_____

NOTES/REMINDERS:

DATE:
/ /

MONDAY

WEEK
12

CARDIOVASCULAR EXERCISE:

EXERCISE TYPE	TIME/DISTANCE/PACE

STRENGTH TRAINING:

EXERCISE TYPE	WEIGHT	SETS	REPS

FLEXIBILITY, RELAXATION MEDITATION:

ACTIVITY PERFORMED	MINUTES

NOTES/REMINDERS:

WEIGHT:

WATER INTAKE:
# of 8oz. glasses
☐ ☐ ☐ ☐
☐ ☐ ☐ ☐

VITAMINS &
SUPPLEMENTS:

ENERGY LEVEL:
☐ low
☐ medium
☐ high

CALORIES
BURNED:

TUESDAY

DATE:
/ /

WEIGHT:

WATER INTAKE:
# of 8oz. glasses
☐ ☐ ☐ ☐
☐ ☐ ☐ ☐

VITAMINS &
SUPPLEMENTS:

ENERGY LEVEL:
☐ low
☐ medium
☐ high

CALORIES
BURNED:

CARDIOVASCULAR EXERCISE:

EXERCISE TYPE	TIME/DISTANCE/PACE

STRENGTH TRAINING:

EXERCISE TYPE	WEIGHT	SETS	REPS

FLEXIBILITY, RELAXATION MEDITATION:

ACTIVITY PERFORMED	MINUTES

NOTES/REMINDERS:

CARDIOVASCULAR EXERCISE:

EXERCISE TYPE	TIME/DISTANCE/PACE

STRENGTH TRAINING:

EXERCISE TYPE	WEIGHT	SETS	REPS

FLEXIBILITY, RELAXATION MEDITATION:

ACTIVITY PERFORMED	MINUTES

NOTES/REMINDERS:

WEIGHT:

WATER INTAKE:
# of 8oz. glasses
☐ ☐ ☐ ☐
☐ ☐ ☐ ☐

VITAMINS &
SUPPLEMENTS:

ENERGY LEVEL:
☐ low
☐ medium
☐ high

CALORIES
BURNED:

THURSDAY

DATE:
/ /

CARDIOVASCULAR EXERCISE:

WEIGHT:

EXERCISE TYPE	TIME/DISTANCE/PACE

WATER INTAKE:
# of 8oz. glasses
☐ ☐ ☐ ☐
☐ ☐ ☐ ☐

STRENGTH TRAINING:

VITAMINS &
SUPPLEMENTS:

EXERCISE TYPE	WEIGHT	SETS	REPS

FLEXIBILITY, RELAXATION MEDITATION:

ACTIVITY PERFORMED	MINUTES

ENERGY LEVEL:
☐ low
☐ medium
☐ high

NOTES/REMINDERS:

CALORIES
BURNED:

FRIDAY

CARDIOVASCULAR EXERCISE:

EXERCISE TYPE	TIME/DISTANCE/PACE

STRENGTH TRAINING:

EXERCISE TYPE	WEIGHT	SETS	REPS

FLEXIBILITY, RELAXATION MEDITATION:

ACTIVITY PERFORMED	MINUTES

NOTES/REMINDERS:

WEIGHT:

WATER INTAKE:
# of 8oz. glasses
☐ ☐ ☐ ☐
☐ ☐ ☐ ☐

VITAMINS & SUPPLEMENTS:

ENERGY LEVEL:
☐ low
☐ medium
☐ high

CALORIES BURNED:

SATURDAY

DATE: / /

WEIGHT:

WATER INTAKE:
# of 8oz. glasses
☐ ☐ ☐ ☐
☐ ☐ ☐ ☐

VITAMINS & SUPPLEMENTS:

_____

_____

_____

_____

_____

_____

_____

ENERGY LEVEL:
☐ low
☐ medium
☐ high

CALORIES BURNED:

CARDIOVASCULAR EXERCISE:

EXERCISE TYPE	TIME/DISTANCE/PACE

STRENGTH TRAINING:

EXERCISE TYPE	WEIGHT	SETS	REPS

FLEXIBILITY, RELAXATION MEDITATION:

ACTIVITY PERFORMED	MINUTES

NOTES/REMINDERS:

DATE:
/ /

SUNDAY

CARDIOVASCULAR EXERCISE:

EXERCISE TYPE	TIME/DISTANCE/PACE

STRENGTH TRAINING:

EXERCISE TYPE	WEIGHT	SETS	REPS

FLEXIBILITY, RELAXATION MEDITATION:

ACTIVITY PERFORMED	MINUTES

NOTES/REMINDERS:

WEIGHT:

WATER INTAKE:
# of 8oz. glasses
☐ ☐ ☐ ☐
☐ ☐ ☐ ☐

VITAMINS &
SUPPLEMENTS:

ENERGY LEVEL:
☐ low
☐ medium
☐ high

CALORIES
BURNED:

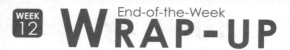

End-of-the-Week

WRAP-UP

WEEKLY ENERGY LEVEL:	START WEIGHT:	END WEIGHT:	WEEKLY CALORIE BURNED:

☐ low ☐ med ☐ high

DAYS I WORKED OUT:

☐ Mon. ☐ Tues. ☐ Wed. ☐ Thurs. ☐ Fri. ☐ Sat. ☐ Sun.

HOW I FELT THIS WEEK:

_____

_____

_____

_____

_____

GOALS FOR NEXT WEEK:

_____

_____

_____

_____

_____

NOTES/REMINDERS:

MONDAY

CARDIOVASCULAR EXERCISE:

EXERCISE TYPE	TIME/DISTANCE/PACE

STRENGTH TRAINING:

EXERCISE TYPE	WEIGHT	SETS	REPS

FLEXIBILITY, RELAXATION MEDITATION:

ACTIVITY PERFORMED	MINUTES

NOTES/REMINDERS:

WEIGHT:

WATER INTAKE:
# of 8oz. glasses
☐ ☐ ☐ ☐
☐ ☐ ☐ ☐

VITAMINS & SUPPLEMENTS:

ENERGY LEVEL:
☐ low
☐ medium
☐ high

CALORIES BURNED:

TUESDAY

DATE:
/ /

WEIGHT:

WATER INTAKE:
# of 8oz. glasses
☐ ☐ ☐ ☐
☐ ☐ ☐ ☐

**VITAMINS &
SUPPLEMENTS:**

ENERGY LEVEL:
☐ low
☐ medium
☐ high

**CALORIES
BURNED:**

CARDIOVASCULAR EXERCISE:

EXERCISE TYPE	TIME/DISTANCE/PACE

STRENGTH TRAINING:

EXERCISE TYPE	WEIGHT	SETS	REPS

FLEXIBILITY, RELAXATION MEDITATION:

ACTIVITY PERFORMED	MINUTES

NOTES/REMINDERS:

DATE:

/ / # **WEDNESDAY**

CARDIOVASCULAR EXERCISE:

EXERCISE TYPE	TIME/DISTANCE/PACE

STRENGTH TRAINING:

EXERCISE TYPE	WEIGHT	SETS	REPS

FLEXIBILITY, RELAXATION MEDITATION:

ACTIVITY PERFORMED	MINUTES

NOTES/REMINDERS:

WEIGHT:

WATER INTAKE:
# of 8oz. glasses
☐ ☐ ☐ ☐
☐ ☐ ☐ ☐

VITAMINS & SUPPLEMENTS:

ENERGY LEVEL:
☐ low
☐ medium
☐ high

CALORIES BURNED:

THURSDAY

DATE:
/ /

WEIGHT:

WATER INTAKE:
# of 8oz. glasses
☐ ☐ ☐ ☐
☐ ☐ ☐ ☐

VITAMINS & SUPPLEMENTS:

_____

_____

_____

_____

_____

_____

_____

ENERGY LEVEL:
☐ low
☐ medium
☐ high

CALORIES BURNED:

CARDIOVASCULAR EXERCISE:

EXERCISE TYPE	TIME/DISTANCE/PACE

STRENGTH TRAINING:

EXERCISE TYPE	WEIGHT	SETS	REPS

FLEXIBILITY, RELAXATION MEDITATION:

ACTIVITY PERFORMED	MINUTES

NOTES/REMINDERS:

DATE:
/ /

FRIDAY

CARDIOVASCULAR EXERCISE:

EXERCISE TYPE	TIME/DISTANCE/PACE

STRENGTH TRAINING:

EXERCISE TYPE	WEIGHT	SETS	REPS

FLEXIBILITY, RELAXATION MEDITATION:

ACTIVITY PERFORMED	MINUTES

NOTES/REMINDERS:

WEIGHT:

WATER INTAKE:
# of 8oz. glasses
☐ ☐ ☐ ☐
☐ ☐ ☐ ☐

VITAMINS & SUPPLEMENTS:

ENERGY LEVEL:
☐ low
☐ medium
☐ high

CALORIES BURNED:

SATURDAY

DATE: / /

WEIGHT:

WATER INTAKE:
# of 8oz. glasses
☐ ☐ ☐ ☐
☐ ☐ ☐ ☐

VITAMINS & SUPPLEMENTS:

ENERGY LEVEL:
☐ low
☐ medium
☐ high

CALORIES BURNED:

CARDIOVASCULAR EXERCISE:

EXERCISE TYPE	TIME/DISTANCE/PACE

STRENGTH TRAINING:

EXERCISE TYPE	WEIGHT	SETS	REPS

FLEXIBILITY, RELAXATION MEDITATION:

ACTIVITY PERFORMED	MINUTES

NOTES/REMINDERS:

DATE: / /

SUNDAY

CARDIOVASCULAR EXERCISE:

EXERCISE TYPE	TIME/DISTANCE/PACE

STRENGTH TRAINING:

EXERCISE TYPE	WEIGHT	SETS	REPS

FLEXIBILITY, RELAXATION MEDITATION:

ACTIVITY PERFORMED	MINUTES

NOTES/REMINDERS:

WEIGHT:

WATER INTAKE:
# of 8oz. glasses
☐ ☐ ☐ ☐
☐ ☐ ☐ ☐

VITAMINS &
SUPPLEMENTS:

ENERGY LEVEL:
☐ low
☐ medium
☐ high

CALORIES
BURNED:

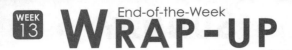

WEEKLY ENERGY LEVEL:	START WEIGHT:	END WEIGHT:	WEEKLY CALORIES BURNED:

☐ low ☐ med ☐ high

DAYS I WORKED OUT:

☐ Mon. ☐ Tues. ☐ Wed. ☐ Thurs. ☐ Fri. ☐ Sat. ☐ Sun.

HOW I FELT THIS WEEK:

_____

_____

_____

_____

_____

GOALS FOR NEXT WEEK:

_____

_____

_____

_____

_____

NOTES/REMINDERS:

DATE:

___ / ___ / ___

MONDAY

CARDIOVASCULAR EXERCISE:

EXERCISE TYPE	TIME/DISTANCE/PACE

STRENGTH TRAINING:

EXERCISE TYPE	WEIGHT	SETS	REPS

FLEXIBILITY, RELAXATION MEDITATION:

ACTIVITY PERFORMED	MINUTES

NOTES/REMINDERS:

WEIGHT:

WATER INTAKE:
# of 8oz. glasses
☐ ☐ ☐ ☐
☐ ☐ ☐ ☐

VITAMINS & SUPPLEMENTS:

ENERGY LEVEL:
☐ low
☐ medium
☐ high

CALORIES BURNED:

TUESDAY

DATE:
/ /

WEIGHT:

WATER INTAKE:
# of 8oz. glasses
☐ ☐ ☐ ☐
☐ ☐ ☐ ☐

**VITAMINS &
SUPPLEMENTS:**

_____

_____

_____

_____

_____

_____

_____

ENERGY LEVEL:
☐ low
☐ medium
☐ high

**CALORIES
BURNED:**

CARDIOVASCULAR EXERCISE:

EXERCISE TYPE	TIME/DISTANCE/PACE

STRENGTH TRAINING:

EXERCISE TYPE	WEIGHT	SETS	REPS

FLEXIBILITY, RELAXATION MEDITATION:

ACTIVITY PERFORMED	MINUTES

NOTES/REMINDERS:

WEDNESDAY

CARDIOVASCULAR EXERCISE:

EXERCISE TYPE	TIME/DISTANCE/PACE

STRENGTH TRAINING:

EXERCISE TYPE	WEIGHT	SETS	REPS

FLEXIBILITY, RELAXATION MEDITATION:

ACTIVITY PERFORMED	MINUTES

NOTES/REMINDERS:

WEIGHT:

WATER INTAKE:
# of 8oz. glasses
☐ ☐ ☐ ☐
☐ ☐ ☐ ☐

VITAMINS & SUPPLEMENTS:

ENERGY LEVEL:
☐ low
☐ medium
☐ high

CALORIES BURNED:

THURSDAY

DATE: / /

WEIGHT:

WATER INTAKE:
# of 8oz. glasses
☐ ☐ ☐ ☐
☐ ☐ ☐ ☐

VITAMINS & SUPPLEMENTS:

ENERGY LEVEL:
☐ low
☐ medium
☐ high

CALORIES BURNED:

CARDIOVASCULAR EXERCISE:

EXERCISE TYPE	TIME/DISTANCE/PACE

STRENGTH TRAINING:

EXERCISE TYPE	WEIGHT	SETS	REPS

FLEXIBILITY, RELAXATION MEDITATION:

ACTIVITY PERFORMED	MINUTES

NOTES/REMINDERS:

FRIDAY

CARDIOVASCULAR EXERCISE:

EXERCISE TYPE	TIME/DISTANCE/PACE

STRENGTH TRAINING:

EXERCISE TYPE	WEIGHT	SETS	REPS

FLEXIBILITY, RELAXATION MEDITATION:

ACTIVITY PERFORMED	MINUTES

NOTES/REMINDERS:

WEIGHT:

WATER INTAKE:
# of 8oz. glasses
☐ ☐ ☐ ☐
☐ ☐ ☐ ☐

VITAMINS & SUPPLEMENTS:

ENERGY LEVEL:
☐ low
☐ medium
☐ high

CALORIES BURNED:

SATURDAY

DATE: ___/___/___

WEIGHT:

WATER INTAKE:
# of 8oz. glasses
☐ ☐ ☐ ☐
☐ ☐ ☐ ☐

VITAMINS & SUPPLEMENTS:

_____
_____
_____
_____
_____
_____
_____

ENERGY LEVEL:
☐ low
☐ medium
☐ high

CALORIES BURNED:

CARDIOVASCULAR EXERCISE:

EXERCISE TYPE	TIME/DISTANCE/PACE

STRENGTH TRAINING:

EXERCISE TYPE	WEIGHT	SETS	REPS

FLEXIBILITY, RELAXATION MEDITATION:

ACTIVITY PERFORMED	MINUTES

NOTES/REMINDERS:

CARDIOVASCULAR EXERCISE:

EXERCISE TYPE	TIME/DISTANCE/PACE

STRENGTH TRAINING:

EXERCISE TYPE	WEIGHT	SETS	REPS

FLEXIBILITY, RELAXATION MEDITATION:

ACTIVITY PERFORMED	MINUTES

NOTES/REMINDERS:

WEIGHT:

WATER INTAKE:
# of 8oz. glasses
☐ ☐ ☐ ☐
☐ ☐ ☐ ☐

VITAMINS & SUPPLEMENTS:

ENERGY LEVEL:
☐ low
☐ medium
☐ high

CALORIES BURNED:

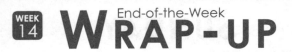

WEEK 14
End-of-the-Week WRAP-UP

WEEKLY ENERGY LEVEL:	START WEIGHT:	END WEIGHT:	WEEKLY CALORIES BURNED:
☐ low ☐ med ☐ high			

DAYS I WORKED OUT:

☐ Mon. ☐ Tues. ☐ Wed. ☐ Thurs. ☐ Fri. ☐ Sat. ☐ Sun.

HOW I FELT THIS WEEK:

_____

_____

_____

_____

_____

GOALS FOR NEXT WEEK:

_____

_____

_____

_____

_____

NOTES/REMINDERS:

DATE:

MONDAY

/ /

CARDIOVASCULAR EXERCISE:

EXERCISE TYPE	TIME/DISTANCE/PACE

STRENGTH TRAINING:

EXERCISE TYPE	WEIGHT	SETS	REPS

FLEXIBILITY, RELAXATION MEDITATION:

ACTIVITY PERFORMED	MINUTES

NOTES/REMINDERS:

WEIGHT:

WATER INTAKE:
# of 8oz. glasses
☐ ☐ ☐ ☐
☐ ☐ ☐ ☐

VITAMINS &
SUPPLEMENTS:

ENERGY LEVEL:
☐ low
☐ medium
☐ high

CALORIES
BURNED:

TUESDAY

DATE: / /

WEIGHT:

WATER INTAKE:
# of 8oz. glasses
☐ ☐ ☐ ☐
☐ ☐ ☐ ☐

VITAMINS & SUPPLEMENTS:

_____

_____

_____

_____

_____

_____

_____

ENERGY LEVEL:
☐ low
☐ medium
☐ high

CALORIES BURNED:

CARDIOVASCULAR EXERCISE:

EXERCISE TYPE	TIME/DISTANCE/PACE

STRENGTH TRAINING:

EXERCISE TYPE	WEIGHT	SETS	REPS

FLEXIBILITY, RELAXATION MEDITATION:

ACTIVITY PERFORMED	MINUTES

NOTES/REMINDERS:

CARDIOVASCULAR EXERCISE:

EXERCISE TYPE	TIME/DISTANCE/PACE

STRENGTH TRAINING:

EXERCISE TYPE	WEIGHT	SETS	REPS

FLEXIBILITY, RELAXATION MEDITATION:

ACTIVITY PERFORMED	MINUTES

NOTES/REMINDERS:

WEIGHT:

WATER INTAKE:
# of 8oz. glasses
☐ ☐ ☐ ☐
☐ ☐ ☐ ☐

VITAMINS & SUPPLEMENTS:

ENERGY LEVEL:
☐ low
☐ medium
☐ high

CALORIES BURNED:

THURSDAY

DATE: / /

WEIGHT:

WATER INTAKE:
# of 8oz. glasses
☐ ☐ ☐ ☐
☐ ☐ ☐ ☐

VITAMINS & SUPPLEMENTS:

ENERGY LEVEL:
☐ low
☐ medium
☐ high

CALORIES BURNED:

CARDIOVASCULAR EXERCISE:

EXERCISE TYPE	TIME/DISTANCE/PACE

STRENGTH TRAINING:

EXERCISE TYPE	WEIGHT	SETS	REPS

FLEXIBILITY, RELAXATION MEDITATION:

ACTIVITY PERFORMED	MINUTES

NOTES/REMINDERS:

CARDIOVASCULAR EXERCISE:

EXERCISE TYPE | TIME/DISTANCE/PACE

WEIGHT:

WATER INTAKE:
# of 8oz. glasses
☐ ☐ ☐ ☐
☐ ☐ ☐ ☐

STRENGTH TRAINING:

EXERCISE TYPE | WEIGHT | SETS | REPS

VITAMINS &
SUPPLEMENTS:

FLEXIBILITY, RELAXATION MEDITATION:

ACTIVITY PERFORMED | MINUTES

ENERGY LEVEL:
☐ low
☐ medium
☐ high

NOTES/REMINDERS:

CALORIES
BURNED:

SATURDAY

DATE: / /

WEIGHT:

WATER INTAKE:
# of 8oz. glasses
☐ ☐ ☐ ☐
☐ ☐ ☐ ☐

VITAMINS & SUPPLEMENTS:

_____
_____
_____
_____
_____
_____
_____
_____

ENERGY LEVEL:
☐ low
☐ medium
☐ high

CALORIES BURNED:

CARDIOVASCULAR EXERCISE:

EXERCISE TYPE	TIME/DISTANCE/PACE

STRENGTH TRAINING:

EXERCISE TYPE	WEIGHT	SETS	REPS

FLEXIBILITY, RELAXATION MEDITATION:

ACTIVITY PERFORMED	MINUTES

NOTES/REMINDERS:

DATE:

/ /

SUNDAY

CARDIOVASCULAR EXERCISE:

EXERCISE TYPE	TIME/DISTANCE/PACE

STRENGTH TRAINING:

EXERCISE TYPE	WEIGHT	SETS	REPS

FLEXIBILITY, RELAXATION MEDITATION:

ACTIVITY PERFORMED	MINUTES

NOTES/REMINDERS:

WEIGHT:

WATER INTAKE:
# of 8oz. glasses
☐ ☐ ☐ ☐
☐ ☐ ☐ ☐

VITAMINS &
SUPPLEMENTS:

ENERGY LEVEL:
☐ low
☐ medium
☐ high

CALORIES
BURNED:

End-of-the-Week
WRAP-UP

WEEKLY ENERGY LEVEL:

☐ low ☐ med ☐ high

START WEIGHT:

END WEIGHT:

WEEKLY CALORIES BURNED:

DAYS I WORKED OUT:

☐ Mon. ☐ Tues. ☐ Wed. ☐ Thurs. ☐ Fri. ☐ Sat. ☐ Sun.

HOW I FELT THIS WEEK:

_____

_____

_____

_____

GOALS FOR NEXT WEEK:

_____

_____

_____

_____

_____

NOTES/REMINDERS:

MONDAY

CARDIOVASCULAR EXERCISE:

EXERCISE TYPE	TIME/DISTANCE/PACE

STRENGTH TRAINING:

EXERCISE TYPE	WEIGHT	SETS	REPS

FLEXIBILITY, RELAXATION MEDITATION:

ACTIVITY PERFORMED	MINUTES

NOTES/REMINDERS:

WEIGHT:

WATER INTAKE:
# of 8oz. glasses
☐ ☐ ☐ ☐
☐ ☐ ☐ ☐

**VITAMINS &
SUPPLEMENTS:**

ENERGY LEVEL:
☐ low
☐ medium
☐ high

**CALORIES
BURNED:**

TUESDAY

DATE: / /

WEIGHT:

WATER INTAKE:
# of 8oz. glasses
☐ ☐ ☐ ☐
☐ ☐ ☐ ☐

VITAMINS & SUPPLEMENTS:

_____
_____
_____
_____
_____
_____
_____

ENERGY LEVEL:
☐ low
☐ medium
☐ high

CALORIES BURNED:

CARDIOVASCULAR EXERCISE:

EXERCISE TYPE	TIME/DISTANCE/PACE

STRENGTH TRAINING:

EXERCISE TYPE	WEIGHT	SETS	REPS

FLEXIBILITY, RELAXATION MEDITATION:

ACTIVITY PERFORMED	MINUTES

NOTES/REMINDERS:

WEDNESDAY

CARDIOVASCULAR EXERCISE:

EXERCISE TYPE	TIME/DISTANCE/PACE

WEIGHT:

WATER INTAKE:
# of 8oz. glasses
☐ ☐ ☐ ☐
☐ ☐ ☐ ☐

STRENGTH TRAINING:

EXERCISE TYPE	WEIGHT	SETS	REPS

VITAMINS & SUPPLEMENTS:

FLEXIBILITY, RELAXATION MEDITATION:

ACTIVITY PERFORMED	MINUTES

ENERGY LEVEL:
☐ low
☐ medium
☐ high

NOTES/REMINDERS:

CALORIES BURNED:

THURSDAY

DATE: ___/___/___

WEIGHT:

WATER INTAKE:
# of 8oz. glasses
☐ ☐ ☐ ☐
☐ ☐ ☐ ☐

VITAMINS & SUPPLEMENTS:

_____
_____
_____
_____
_____
_____
_____

ENERGY LEVEL:
☐ low
☐ medium
☐ high

CALORIES BURNED:

CARDIOVASCULAR EXERCISE:

EXERCISE TYPE	TIME/DISTANCE/PACE

STRENGTH TRAINING:

EXERCISE TYPE	WEIGHT	SETS	REPS

FLEXIBILITY, RELAXATION MEDITATION:

ACTIVITY PERFORMED	MINUTES

NOTES/REMINDERS:

DATE:
/ /

FRIDAY

CARDIOVASCULAR EXERCISE:

EXERCISE TYPE   **TIME/DISTANCE/PACE**

_____   _____

_____   _____

_____   _____

STRENGTH TRAINING:

EXERCISE TYPE   **WEIGHT** **SETS** **REPS**

FLEXIBILITY, RELAXATION MEDITATION:

ACTIVITY PERFORMED   **MINUTES**

_____   _____

_____   _____

_____   _____

NOTES/REMINDERS:

WEIGHT:

WATER INTAKE:
# of 8oz. glasses
☐ ☐ ☐ ☐
☐ ☐ ☐ ☐

**VITAMINS &
SUPPLEMENTS:**

ENERGY LEVEL:
☐ low
☐ medium
☐ high

**CALORIES
BURNED:**

WEEK 16

SATURDAY

DATE: / /

WEIGHT:

WATER INTAKE:
# of 8oz. glasses
☐ ☐ ☐ ☐
☐ ☐ ☐ ☐

**VITAMINS &
SUPPLEMENTS:**

_____

_____

_____

_____

_____

_____

_____

ENERGY LEVEL:
☐ low
☐ medium
☐ high

**CALORIES
BURNED:**

CARDIOVASCULAR EXERCISE:

EXERCISE TYPE	TIME/DISTANCE/PACE

STRENGTH TRAINING:

EXERCISE TYPE	WEIGHT	SETS	REPS

FLEXIBILITY, RELAXATION MEDITATION:

ACTIVITY PERFORMED	MINUTES

NOTES/REMINDERS:

DATE:
/ /

SUNDAY

CARDIOVASCULAR EXERCISE:

EXERCISE TYPE	TIME/DISTANCE/PACE

STRENGTH TRAINING:

EXERCISE TYPE	WEIGHT	SETS	REPS

FLEXIBILITY, RELAXATION MEDITATION:

ACTIVITY PERFORMED	MINUTES

NOTES/REMINDERS:

WEIGHT:

WATER INTAKE:
# of 8oz. glasses
☐ ☐ ☐ ☐
☐ ☐ ☐ ☐

VITAMINS & SUPPLEMENTS:

ENERGY LEVEL:
☐ low
☐ medium
☐ high

CALORIES BURNED:

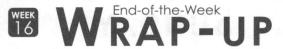

| WEEKLY ENERGY LEVEL: | START WEIGHT: | END WEIGHT: | WEEKLY CALORIES BURNED: |

☐ low ☐ med ☐ high

DAYS I WORKED OUT:

☐ Mon. ☐ Tues. ☐ Wed. ☐ Thurs. ☐ Fri. ☐ Sat. ☐ Sun.

HOW I FELT THIS WEEK:

_____

_____

_____

_____

_____

GOALS FOR NEXT WEEK:

_____

_____

_____

_____

_____

NOTES/REMINDERS:

DATE:
/ /

MONDAY

CARDIOVASCULAR EXERCISE:

EXERCISE TYPE　　　　　　　　　**TIME/DISTANCE/PACE**

WEIGHT:

WATER INTAKE:
# of 8oz. glasses
☐ ☐ ☐ ☐
☐ ☐ ☐ ☐

STRENGTH TRAINING:

EXERCISE TYPE　　　　　**WEIGHT SETS REPS**

**VITAMINS &
SUPPLEMENTS:**

FLEXIBILITY, RELAXATION MEDITATION:

ACTIVITY PERFORMED　　　　　**MINUTES**

ENERGY LEVEL:
☐ low
☐ medium
☐ high

NOTES/REMINDERS:

**CALORIES
BURNED:**

TUESDAY

DATE: _ / _ / _

WEIGHT:

WATER INTAKE:
# of 8oz. glasses
☐ ☐ ☐ ☐
☐ ☐ ☐ ☐

**VITAMINS &
SUPPLEMENTS:**

_____

_____

_____

_____

_____

_____

_____

ENERGY LEVEL:
☐ low
☐ medium
☐ high

**CALORIES
BURNED:**

CARDIOVASCULAR EXERCISE:

EXERCISE TYPE	TIME/DISTANCE/PACE

STRENGTH TRAINING:

EXERCISE TYPE	WEIGHT	SETS	REPS

FLEXIBILITY, RELAXATION MEDITATION:

ACTIVITY PERFORMED	MINUTES

NOTES/REMINDERS:

CARDIOVASCULAR EXERCISE:

EXERCISE TYPE	TIME/DISTANCE/PACE

STRENGTH TRAINING:

EXERCISE TYPE	WEIGHT	SETS	REPS

FLEXIBILITY, RELAXATION MEDITATION:

ACTIVITY PERFORMED	MINUTES

NOTES/REMINDERS:

WEIGHT:

WATER INTAKE:
# of 8oz. glasses
☐ ☐ ☐ ☐
☐ ☐ ☐ ☐

VITAMINS & SUPPLEMENTS:

ENERGY LEVEL:
☐ low
☐ medium
☐ high

CALORIES BURNED:

THURSDAY

DATE: / /

WEIGHT:

WATER INTAKE:
# of 8oz. glasses
☐ ☐ ☐ ☐
☐ ☐ ☐ ☐

VITAMINS & SUPPLEMENTS:

ENERGY LEVEL:
☐ low
☐ medium
☐ high

CALORIES BURNED:

CARDIOVASCULAR EXERCISE:

EXERCISE TYPE	TIME/DISTANCE/PACE

STRENGTH TRAINING:

EXERCISE TYPE	WEIGHT	SETS	REPS

FLEXIBILITY, RELAXATION MEDITATION:

ACTIVITY PERFORMED	MINUTES

NOTES/REMINDERS:

DATE:
/ /

FRIDAY

CARDIOVASCULAR EXERCISE:

EXERCISE TYPE	TIME/DISTANCE/PACE

STRENGTH TRAINING:

EXERCISE TYPE	WEIGHT	SETS	REPS

FLEXIBILITY, RELAXATION MEDITATION:

ACTIVITY PERFORMED	MINUTES

NOTES/REMINDERS:

WEIGHT:

WATER INTAKE:
# of 8oz. glasses
☐ ☐ ☐ ☐
☐ ☐ ☐ ☐

VITAMINS & SUPPLEMENTS:

ENERGY LEVEL:
☐ low
☐ medium
☐ high

CALORIES BURNED:

SATURDAY

DATE: __ / __ / __

WEIGHT:

WATER INTAKE:
# of 8oz. glasses
☐ ☐ ☐ ☐
☐ ☐ ☐ ☐

VITAMINS & SUPPLEMENTS:

_____
_____
_____
_____
_____
_____
_____
_____

ENERGY LEVEL:
☐ low
☐ medium
☐ high

CALORIES BURNED:

CARDIOVASCULAR EXERCISE:

EXERCISE TYPE	TIME/DISTANCE/PACE

STRENGTH TRAINING:

EXERCISE TYPE	WEIGHT	SETS	REPS

FLEXIBILITY, RELAXATION MEDITATION:

ACTIVITY PERFORMED	MINUTES

NOTES/REMINDERS:

DATE:

/ /

SUNDAY

CARDIOVASCULAR EXERCISE:

EXERCISE TYPE	TIME/DISTANCE/PACE

WEIGHT:

WATER INTAKE:
# of 8oz. glasses
☐ ☐ ☐ ☐
☐ ☐ ☐ ☐

STRENGTH TRAINING:

EXERCISE TYPE	WEIGHT	SETS	REPS

**VITAMINS &
SUPPLEMENTS:**

FLEXIBILITY, RELAXATION MEDITATION:

ACTIVITY PERFORMED	MINUTES

ENERGY LEVEL:
☐ low
☐ medium
☐ high

NOTES/REMINDERS:

**CALORIES
BURNED:**

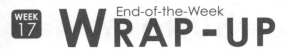

WRAP-UP
End-of-the-Week

WEEKLY ENERGY LEVEL: **START WEIGHT:** **END WEIGHT:** **WEEKLY CALORIES BURNED:**

☐ low ☐ med ☐ high

DAYS I WORKED OUT:

☐ Mon. ☐ Tues. ☐ Wed. ☐ Thurs. ☐ Fri. ☐ Sat. ☐ Sun.

HOW I FELT THIS WEEK:

_____

_____

_____

_____

_____

GOALS FOR NEXT WEEK:

_____

_____

_____

_____

_____

NOTES/REMINDERS:

DATE:
/ /

MONDAY

CARDIOVASCULAR EXERCISE:

EXERCISE TYPE	TIME/DISTANCE/PACE

STRENGTH TRAINING:

EXERCISE TYPE	WEIGHT	SETS	REPS

FLEXIBILITY, RELAXATION MEDITATION:

ACTIVITY PERFORMED	MINUTES

NOTES/REMINDERS:

WEIGHT:

WATER INTAKE:
# of 8oz. glasses
☐ ☐ ☐ ☐
☐ ☐ ☐ ☐

VITAMINS & SUPPLEMENTS:

ENERGY LEVEL:
☐ low
☐ medium
☐ high

CALORIES BURNED:

TUESDAY

DATE:
/ /

WEIGHT:

WATER INTAKE:
# of 8oz. glasses
☐ ☐ ☐ ☐
☐ ☐ ☐ ☐

VITAMINS & SUPPLEMENTS:

_____
_____
_____
_____
_____
_____
_____
_____

ENERGY LEVEL:
☐ low
☐ medium
☐ high

CALORIES BURNED:

CARDIOVASCULAR EXERCISE:

EXERCISE TYPE	TIME/DISTANCE/PACE

STRENGTH TRAINING:

EXERCISE TYPE	WEIGHT	SETS	REPS

FLEXIBILITY, RELAXATION MEDITATION:

ACTIVITY PERFORMED	MINUTES

NOTES/REMINDERS:

DATE:
/ /

WEDNESDAY

WEEK 18

CARDIOVASCULAR EXERCISE:

EXERCISE TYPE	TIME/DISTANCE/PACE

STRENGTH TRAINING:

EXERCISE TYPE	WEIGHT	SETS	REPS

FLEXIBILITY, RELAXATION MEDITATION:

ACTIVITY PERFORMED	MINUTES

NOTES/REMINDERS:

WEIGHT:

WATER INTAKE:
# of 8oz. glasses
☐ ☐ ☐ ☐
☐ ☐ ☐ ☐

VITAMINS & SUPPLEMENTS:

ENERGY LEVEL:
☐ low
☐ medium
☐ high

CALORIES BURNED:

THURSDAY

DATE: / /

WEIGHT:

WATER INTAKE:
# of 8oz. glasses
☐ ☐ ☐ ☐
☐ ☐ ☐ ☐

VITAMINS & SUPPLEMENTS:

_____

_____

_____

_____

_____

_____

_____

ENERGY LEVEL:
☐ low
☐ medium
☐ high

CALORIES BURNED:

CARDIOVASCULAR EXERCISE:

EXERCISE TYPE	TIME/DISTANCE/PACE

STRENGTH TRAINING:

EXERCISE TYPE	WEIGHT	SETS	REPS

FLEXIBILITY, RELAXATION MEDITATION:

ACTIVITY PERFORMED	MINUTES

NOTES/REMINDERS:

DATE:
/ /

FRIDAY

CARDIOVASCULAR EXERCISE:

EXERCISE TYPE	TIME/DISTANCE/PACE

STRENGTH TRAINING:

EXERCISE TYPE	WEIGHT	SETS	REPS

FLEXIBILITY, RELAXATION MEDITATION:

ACTIVITY PERFORMED	MINUTES

NOTES/REMINDERS:

WEIGHT:

WATER INTAKE:
# of 8oz. glasses
☐ ☐ ☐ ☐
☐ ☐ ☐ ☐

VITAMINS & SUPPLEMENTS:

ENERGY LEVEL:
☐ low
☐ medium
☐ high

CALORIES BURNED:

SATURDAY

DATE: / /

WEIGHT:

WATER INTAKE:
# of 8oz. glasses
☐ ☐ ☐ ☐
☐ ☐ ☐ ☐

VITAMINS & SUPPLEMENTS:

_____

_____

_____

_____

_____

_____

_____

ENERGY LEVEL:
☐ low
☐ medium
☐ high

CALORIES BURNED:

CARDIOVASCULAR EXERCISE:

EXERCISE TYPE	TIME/DISTANCE/PACE

STRENGTH TRAINING:

EXERCISE TYPE	WEIGHT	SETS	REPS

FLEXIBILITY, RELAXATION MEDITATION:

ACTIVITY PERFORMED	MINUTES

NOTES/REMINDERS:

DATE:
/ /

SUNDAY

CARDIOVASCULAR EXERCISE:

EXERCISE TYPE	TIME/DISTANCE/PACE

STRENGTH TRAINING:

EXERCISE TYPE	WEIGHT	SETS	REPS

FLEXIBILITY, RELAXATION MEDITATION:

ACTIVITY PERFORMED	MINUTES

NOTES/REMINDERS:

WEIGHT:

WATER INTAKE:
# of 8oz. glasses
☐ ☐ ☐ ☐
☐ ☐ ☐ ☐

VITAMINS & SUPPLEMENTS:

ENERGY LEVEL:
☐ low
☐ medium
☐ high

CALORIES BURNED:

End-of-the-Week WRAP-UP

WEEKLY ENERGY LEVEL:	START WEIGHT:	END WEIGHT:	WEEKLY CALORIES BURNED:
☐ low ☐ med ☐ high			

DAYS I WORKED OUT:
☐ Mon. ☐ Tues. ☐ Wed. ☐ Thurs. ☐ Fri. ☐ Sat. ☐ Sun.

HOW I FELT THIS WEEK:

_____

_____

_____

_____

_____

GOALS FOR NEXT WEEK:

_____

_____

_____

_____

_____

NOTES/REMINDERS:

CARDIOVASCULAR EXERCISE:

EXERCISE TYPE	TIME/DISTANCE/PACE

STRENGTH TRAINING:

EXERCISE TYPE	WEIGHT	SETS	REPS

FLEXIBILITY, RELAXATION MEDITATION:

ACTIVITY PERFORMED	MINUTES

NOTES/REMINDERS:

WEIGHT:

WATER INTAKE:
# of 8oz. glasses
☐ ☐ ☐ ☐
☐ ☐ ☐ ☐

VITAMINS &
SUPPLEMENTS:

ENERGY LEVEL:
☐ low
☐ medium
☐ high

CALORIES
BURNED:

TUESDAY

DATE: / /

WEIGHT:

WATER INTAKE:
# of 8oz. glasses
☐ ☐ ☐ ☐
☐ ☐ ☐ ☐

VITAMINS & SUPPLEMENTS:

ENERGY LEVEL:
☐ low
☐ medium
☐ high

CALORIES BURNED:

CARDIOVASCULAR EXERCISE:

EXERCISE TYPE	TIME/DISTANCE/PACE

STRENGTH TRAINING:

EXERCISE TYPE	WEIGHT	SETS	REPS

FLEXIBILITY, RELAXATION MEDITATION:

ACTIVITY PERFORMED	MINUTES

NOTES/REMINDERS:

WEDNESDAY

CARDIOVASCULAR EXERCISE:

EXERCISE TYPE	TIME/DISTANCE/PACE

STRENGTH TRAINING:

EXERCISE TYPE	WEIGHT	SETS	REPS

FLEXIBILITY, RELAXATION MEDITATION:

ACTIVITY PERFORMED	MINUTES

NOTES/REMINDERS:

WEIGHT:

WATER INTAKE:
# of 8oz. glasses
☐ ☐ ☐ ☐
☐ ☐ ☐ ☐

VITAMINS & SUPPLEMENTS:

ENERGY LEVEL:
☐ low
☐ medium
☐ high

CALORIES BURNED:

THURSDAY

DATE:
/ /

WEIGHT:

WATER INTAKE:
# of 8oz. glasses
☐ ☐ ☐ ☐
☐ ☐ ☐ ☐

VITAMINS & SUPPLEMENTS:

ENERGY LEVEL:
☐ low
☐ medium
☐ high

CALORIES BURNED:

CARDIOVASCULAR EXERCISE:

EXERCISE TYPE	TIME/DISTANCE/PACE

STRENGTH TRAINING:

EXERCISE TYPE	WEIGHT	SETS	REPS

FLEXIBILITY, RELAXATION MEDITATION:

ACTIVITY PERFORMED	MINUTES

NOTES/REMINDERS:

FRIDAY

CARDIOVASCULAR EXERCISE:

EXERCISE TYPE	TIME/DISTANCE/PACE

WEIGHT:

WATER INTAKE:
# of 8oz. glasses
☐ ☐ ☐ ☐
☐ ☐ ☐ ☐

STRENGTH TRAINING:

EXERCISE TYPE	WEIGHT	SETS	REPS

VITAMINS & SUPPLEMENTS:

FLEXIBILITY, RELAXATION MEDITATION:

ACTIVITY PERFORMED	MINUTES

ENERGY LEVEL:
☐ low
☐ medium
☐ high

NOTES/REMINDERS:

CALORIES BURNED:

SATURDAY

DATE: / /

WEIGHT:

WATER INTAKE:
# of 8oz. glasses
☐ ☐ ☐ ☐
☐ ☐ ☐ ☐

VITAMINS & SUPPLEMENTS:

ENERGY LEVEL:
☐ low
☐ medium
☐ high

CALORIES BURNED:

CARDIOVASCULAR EXERCISE:

EXERCISE TYPE	TIME/DISTANCE/PACE

STRENGTH TRAINING:

EXERCISE TYPE	WEIGHT	SETS	REPS

FLEXIBILITY, RELAXATION MEDITATION:

ACTIVITY PERFORMED	MINUTES

NOTES/REMINDERS:

DATE:

/ /

SUNDAY

CARDIOVASCULAR EXERCISE:

EXERCISE TYPE	TIME/DISTANCE/PACE

STRENGTH TRAINING:

EXERCISE TYPE	WEIGHT	SETS	REPS

FLEXIBILITY, RELAXATION MEDITATION:

ACTIVITY PERFORMED	MINUTES

NOTES/REMINDERS:

WEIGHT:

WATER INTAKE:
# of 8oz. glasses
☐ ☐ ☐ ☐
☐ ☐ ☐ ☐

VITAMINS & SUPPLEMENTS:

ENERGY LEVEL:
☐ low
☐ medium
☐ high

CALORIES BURNED:

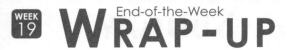

WEEKLY ENERGY LEVEL:

☐ low ☐ med ☐ high

START WEIGHT:

END WEIGHT:

WEEKLY CALORIES BURNED:

DAYS I WORKED OUT:

☐ Mon. ☐ Tues. ☐ Wed. ☐ Thurs. ☐ Fri. ☐ Sat. ☐ Sun.

HOW I FELT THIS WEEK:

_____

_____

_____

_____

GOALS FOR NEXT WEEK:

_____

_____

_____

_____

_____

NOTES/REMINDERS:

DATE:
/ /

MONDAY

CARDIOVASCULAR EXERCISE:

EXERCISE TYPE	TIME/DISTANCE/PACE

STRENGTH TRAINING:

EXERCISE TYPE	WEIGHT	SETS	REPS

FLEXIBILITY, RELAXATION MEDITATION:

ACTIVITY PERFORMED	MINUTES

NOTES/REMINDERS:

WEIGHT:

WATER INTAKE:
# of 8oz. glasses
☐ ☐ ☐ ☐
☐ ☐ ☐ ☐

VITAMINS & SUPPLEMENTS:

ENERGY LEVEL:
☐ low
☐ medium
☐ high

CALORIES BURNED:

TUESDAY

DATE: / /

WEIGHT:

WATER INTAKE:
# of 8oz. glasses
☐ ☐ ☐ ☐
☐ ☐ ☐ ☐

VITAMINS & SUPPLEMENTS:

_____

_____

_____

_____

_____

_____

ENERGY LEVEL:
☐ low
☐ medium
☐ high

CALORIES BURNED:

CARDIOVASCULAR EXERCISE:

EXERCISE TYPE	TIME/DISTANCE/PACE

STRENGTH TRAINING:

EXERCISE TYPE	WEIGHT	SETS	REPS

FLEXIBILITY, RELAXATION MEDITATION:

ACTIVITY PERFORMED	MINUTES

NOTES/REMINDERS:

DATE:

WEDNESDAY

___ / ___ / ___

CARDIOVASCULAR EXERCISE:

EXERCISE TYPE	TIME/DISTANCE/PACE

WEIGHT:

WATER INTAKE:
# of 8oz. glasses
☐ ☐ ☐ ☐
☐ ☐ ☐ ☐

STRENGTH TRAINING:

EXERCISE TYPE	WEIGHT	SETS	REPS

VITAMINS & SUPPLEMENTS:

FLEXIBILITY, RELAXATION MEDITATION:

ACTIVITY PERFORMED	MINUTES

ENERGY LEVEL:
☐ low
☐ medium
☐ high

NOTES/REMINDERS:

CALORIES BURNED:

THURSDAY

DATE: / /

WEIGHT:

CARDIOVASCULAR EXERCISE:

EXERCISE TYPE	TIME/DISTANCE/PACE

WATER INTAKE:
# of 8oz. glasses
☐ ☐ ☐ ☐
☐ ☐ ☐ ☐

VITAMINS & SUPPLEMENTS:

STRENGTH TRAINING:

EXERCISE TYPE	WEIGHT	SETS	REPS

FLEXIBILITY, RELAXATION MEDITATION:

ACTIVITY PERFORMED	MINUTES

ENERGY LEVEL:
☐ low
☐ medium
☐ high

NOTES/REMINDERS:

CALORIES BURNED:

DATE:

/ /

FRIDAY

CARDIOVASCULAR EXERCISE:

EXERCISE TYPE	TIME/DISTANCE/PACE

WEIGHT:

WATER INTAKE:
# of 8oz. glasses
☐ ☐ ☐ ☐
☐ ☐ ☐ ☐

STRENGTH TRAINING:

EXERCISE TYPE	WEIGHT	SETS	REPS

VITAMINS & SUPPLEMENTS:

_____

_____

_____

_____

_____

_____

FLEXIBILITY, RELAXATION MEDITATION:

ACTIVITY PERFORMED	MINUTES

ENERGY LEVEL:
☐ low
☐ medium
☐ high

NOTES/REMINDERS:

CALORIES BURNED:

SATURDAY

DATE:
/ /

WEIGHT:

WATER INTAKE:
# of 8oz. glasses
☐ ☐ ☐ ☐
☐ ☐ ☐ ☐

**VITAMINS &
SUPPLEMENTS:**

ENERGY LEVEL:
☐ low
☐ medium
☐ high

**CALORIES
BURNED:**

CARDIOVASCULAR EXERCISE:

EXERCISE TYPE	TIME/DISTANCE/PACE

STRENGTH TRAINING:

EXERCISE TYPE	WEIGHT	SETS	REPS

FLEXIBILITY, RELAXATION MEDITATION:

ACTIVITY PERFORMED	MINUTES

NOTES/REMINDERS:

DATE:

/ /

SUNDAY

CARDIOVASCULAR EXERCISE:

EXERCISE TYPE

TIME/DISTANCE/PACE

WEIGHT:

WATER INTAKE:
# of 8oz. glasses

☐ ☐ ☐ ☐
☐ ☐ ☐ ☐

STRENGTH TRAINING:

EXERCISE TYPE

WEIGHT **SETS** **REPS**

VITAMINS &
SUPPLEMENTS:

FLEXIBILITY, RELAXATION MEDITATION:

ACTIVITY PERFORMED

MINUTES

ENERGY LEVEL:

☐ low
☐ medium
☐ high

NOTES/REMINDERS:

CALORIES
BURNED:

End-of-the-Week
WRAP-UP

WEEKLY ENERGY LEVEL:	START WEIGHT:	END WEIGHT:	WEEKLY CALORIES BURNED:

☐ low ☐ med ☐ high

DAYS I WORKED OUT:

☐ Mon. ☐ Tues. ☐ Wed. ☐ Thurs. ☐ Fri. ☐ Sat. ☐ Sun.

HOW I FELT THIS WEEK:

_____

_____

_____

_____

_____

GOALS FOR NEXT WEEK:

_____

_____

_____

_____

_____

NOTES/REMINDERS:

DATE:
/ /

MONDAY

CARDIOVASCULAR EXERCISE:

EXERCISE TYPE

TIME/DISTANCE/PACE

STRENGTH TRAINING:

EXERCISE TYPE

WEIGHT **SETS** **REPS**

FLEXIBILITY, RELAXATION MEDITATION:

ACTIVITY PERFORMED

MINUTES

NOTES/REMINDERS:

WEIGHT:

WATER INTAKE:
# of 8oz. glasses
☐ ☐ ☐ ☐
☐ ☐ ☐ ☐

**VITAMINS &
SUPPLEMENTS:**

ENERGY LEVEL:
☐ low
☐ medium
☐ high

**CALORIES
BURNED:**

TUESDAY

DATE: __ / __ / __

WEIGHT:

WATER INTAKE:
# of 8oz. glasses
☐ ☐ ☐
☐ ☐ ☐

VITAMINS & SUPPLEMENTS:

_____

_____

_____

_____

_____

_____

_____

ENERGY LEVEL:
☐ low
☐ medium
☐ high

CALORIES BURNED:

CARDIOVASCULAR EXERCISE:

EXERCISE TYPE	TIME/DISTANCE/PACE

STRENGTH TRAINING:

EXERCISE TYPE	WEIGHT	SETS	REPS

FLEXIBILITY, RELAXATION MEDITATION:

ACTIVITY PERFORMED	MINUTES

NOTES/REMINDERS:

WEDNESDAY

CARDIOVASCULAR EXERCISE:

EXERCISE TYPE	TIME/DISTANCE/PACE

STRENGTH TRAINING:

EXERCISE TYPE	WEIGHT	SETS	REPS

FLEXIBILITY, RELAXATION MEDITATION:

ACTIVITY PERFORMED	MINUTES

NOTES/REMINDERS:

WEIGHT:

WATER INTAKE:
# of 8oz. glasses
☐ ☐ ☐ ☐
☐ ☐ ☐ ☐

VITAMINS & SUPPLEMENTS:

ENERGY LEVEL:
☐ low
☐ medium
☐ high

CALORIES BURNED:

THURSDAY

DATE: __ / __ / __

WEIGHT:

WATER INTAKE:
# of 8oz. glasses
☐ ☐ ☐ ☐
☐ ☐ ☐ ☐

VITAMINS & SUPPLEMENTS:

_____
_____
_____
_____
_____
_____
_____
_____

ENERGY LEVEL:
☐ low
☐ medium
☐ high

CALORIES BURNED:

CARDIOVASCULAR EXERCISE:

EXERCISE TYPE	TIME/DISTANCE/PACE

STRENGTH TRAINING:

EXERCISE TYPE	WEIGHT	SETS	REPS

FLEXIBILITY, RELAXATION MEDITATION:

ACTIVITY PERFORMED	MINUTES

NOTES/REMINDERS:

DATE:

/ /

FRIDAY

CARDIOVASCULAR EXERCISE:

EXERCISE TYPE	TIME/DISTANCE/PACE

STRENGTH TRAINING:

EXERCISE TYPE	WEIGHT	SETS	REPS

FLEXIBILITY, RELAXATION MEDITATION:

ACTIVITY PERFORMED	MINUTES

NOTES/REMINDERS:

WEIGHT:

WATER INTAKE:
# of 8oz. glasses
☐ ☐ ☐ ☐
☐ ☐ ☐ ☐

VITAMINS &
SUPPLEMENTS:

ENERGY LEVEL:
☐ low
☐ medium
☐ high

CALORIES
BURNED:

SATURDAY

DATE: __ / __ / __

WEIGHT:

WATER INTAKE:
# of 8oz. glasses
☐ ☐ ☐ ☐
☐ ☐ ☐ ☐

VITAMINS & SUPPLEMENTS:

ENERGY LEVEL:
☐ low
☐ medium
☐ high

CALORIES BURNED:

CARDIOVASCULAR EXERCISE:

EXERCISE TYPE	TIME/DISTANCE/PACE

STRENGTH TRAINING:

EXERCISE TYPE	WEIGHT	SETS	REPS

FLEXIBILITY, RELAXATION MEDITATION:

ACTIVITY PERFORMED	MINUTES

NOTES/REMINDERS:

DATE:
/ /

SUNDAY

CARDIOVASCULAR EXERCISE:

EXERCISE TYPE	TIME/DISTANCE/PACE

STRENGTH TRAINING:

EXERCISE TYPE	WEIGHT	SETS	REPS

FLEXIBILITY, RELAXATION MEDITATION:

ACTIVITY PERFORMED	MINUTES

NOTES/REMINDERS:

WEIGHT:

WATER INTAKE:
# of 8oz. glasses
☐ ☐ ☐ ☐
☐ ☐ ☐ ☐

VITAMINS &
SUPPLEMENTS:

ENERGY LEVEL:
☐ low
☐ medium
☐ high

CALORIES
BURNED:

End-of-the-Week WRAP-UP

WEEKLY ENERGY LEVEL:	START WEIGHT:	END WEIGHT:	WEEKLY CALORIE BURNED:

☐ low ☐ med ☐ high

DAYS I WORKED OUT:

☐ Mon. ☐ Tues. ☐ Wed. ☐ Thurs. ☐ Fri. ☐ Sat. ☐ Sun.

HOW I FELT THIS WEEK:

_____

_____

_____

_____

_____

GOALS FOR NEXT WEEK:

_____

_____

_____

_____

_____

NOTES/REMINDERS:

DATE:

MONDAY

/ /

CARDIOVASCULAR EXERCISE:

EXERCISE TYPE	TIME/DISTANCE/PACE

STRENGTH TRAINING:

EXERCISE TYPE	WEIGHT	SETS	REPS

FLEXIBILITY, RELAXATION MEDITATION:

ACTIVITY PERFORMED	MINUTES

NOTES/REMINDERS:

WEIGHT:

WATER INTAKE:
# of 8oz. glasses
☐ ☐ ☐ ☐
☐ ☐ ☐ ☐

**VITAMINS &
SUPPLEMENTS:**

ENERGY LEVEL:
☐ low
☐ medium
☐ high

**CALORIES
BURNED:**

WEEK 22

TUESDAY

DATE: _/_/_

WEIGHT:

WATER INTAKE:
# of 8oz. glasses
☐ ☐ ☐ ☐
☐ ☐ ☐ ☐

**VITAMINS &
SUPPLEMENTS:**

_____

_____

_____

_____

_____

_____

_____

ENERGY LEVEL:
☐ low
☐ medium
☐ high

**CALORIES
BURNED:**

CARDIOVASCULAR EXERCISE:

EXERCISE TYPE	TIME/DISTANCE/PACE

STRENGTH TRAINING:

EXERCISE TYPE	WEIGHT	SETS	REPS

FLEXIBILITY, RELAXATION MEDITATION:

ACTIVITY PERFORMED	MINUTES

NOTES/REMINDERS:

DATE:
__/__/__

WEDNESDAY

CARDIOVASCULAR EXERCISE:

EXERCISE TYPE	TIME/DISTANCE/PACE

STRENGTH TRAINING:

EXERCISE TYPE	WEIGHT	SETS	REPS

FLEXIBILITY, RELAXATION MEDITATION:

ACTIVITY PERFORMED	MINUTES

NOTES/REMINDERS:

WEIGHT:

WATER INTAKE:
# of 8oz. glasses
☐ ☐ ☐ ☐
☐ ☐ ☐ ☐

VITAMINS & SUPPLEMENTS:

ENERGY LEVEL:
☐ low
☐ medium
☐ high

CALORIES BURNED:

THURSDAY

DATE: __/__/__

WEIGHT:

WATER INTAKE:
# of 8oz. glasses
☐ ☐ ☐ ☐
☐ ☐ ☐ ☐

VITAMINS & SUPPLEMENTS:

_____
_____
_____
_____
_____
_____
_____

CARDIOVASCULAR EXERCISE:

EXERCISE TYPE	TIME/DISTANCE/PACE

STRENGTH TRAINING:

EXERCISE TYPE	WEIGHT	SETS	REPS

FLEXIBILITY, RELAXATION MEDITATION:

ACTIVITY PERFORMED	MINUTES

ENERGY LEVEL:
☐ low
☐ medium
☐ high

NOTES/REMINDERS:

CALORIES BURNED:

DATE:
/ /

FRIDAY

CARDIOVASCULAR EXERCISE:

EXERCISE TYPE   **TIME/DISTANCE/PACE**

WEIGHT:

WATER INTAKE:
# of 8oz. glasses
☐ ☐ ☐ ☐
☐ ☐ ☐ ☐

STRENGTH TRAINING:

EXERCISE TYPE   **WEIGHT**   **SETS**   **REPS**

VITAMINS &
SUPPLEMENTS:

FLEXIBILITY, RELAXATION MEDITATION:

ACTIVITY PERFORMED   **MINUTES**

ENERGY LEVEL:
☐ low
☐ medium
☐ high

NOTES/REMINDERS:

CALORIES
BURNED:

WEEK 22

SATURDAY

DATE: / /

WEIGHT:

WATER INTAKE:
# of 8oz. glasses
☐ ☐ ☐ ☐
☐ ☐ ☐ ☐

VITAMINS & SUPPLEMENTS:

_____
_____
_____
_____
_____
_____
_____

ENERGY LEVEL:
☐ low
☐ medium
☐ high

CALORIES BURNED:

CARDIOVASCULAR EXERCISE:

EXERCISE TYPE	TIME/DISTANCE/PACE

STRENGTH TRAINING:

EXERCISE TYPE	WEIGHT	SETS	REPS

FLEXIBILITY, RELAXATION MEDITATION:

ACTIVITY PERFORMED	MINUTES

NOTES/REMINDERS:

DATE:
/ /

SUNDAY

CARDIOVASCULAR EXERCISE:

EXERCISE TYPE

TIME/DISTANCE/PACE

_____   _____

_____   _____

_____   _____

STRENGTH TRAINING:

EXERCISE TYPE   **WEIGHT** **SETS** **REPS**

WEIGHT:

WATER INTAKE:
# of 8oz. glasses
☐ ☐ ☐ ☐
☐ ☐ ☐ ☐

**VITAMINS &
SUPPLEMENTS:**

_____

_____

_____

_____

_____

FLEXIBILITY, RELAXATION MEDITATION:

ACTIVITY PERFORMED   **MINUTES**

_____   _____

_____   _____

_____   _____

ENERGY LEVEL:
☐ low
☐ medium
☐ high

NOTES/REMINDERS:

**CALORIES
BURNED:**

End-of-the-Week WRAP-UP

WEEKLY ENERGY LEVEL:

☐ low ☐ med ☐ high

START WEIGHT:

END WEIGHT:

WEEKLY CALORIES BURNED:

DAYS I WORKED OUT:

☐ Mon. ☐ Tues. ☐ Wed. ☐ Thurs. ☐ Fri. ☐ Sat. ☐ Sun.

HOW I FELT THIS WEEK:

_____

_____

_____

_____

_____

GOALS FOR NEXT WEEK:

_____

_____

_____

_____

_____

NOTES/REMINDERS:

DATE:
___/___/___

MONDAY

CARDIOVASCULAR EXERCISE:

EXERCISE TYPE	TIME/DISTANCE/PACE

WEIGHT:

WATER INTAKE:
# of 8oz. glasses
☐ ☐ ☐ ☐
☐ ☐ ☐ ☐

STRENGTH TRAINING:

EXERCISE TYPE	WEIGHT	SETS	REPS

VITAMINS & SUPPLEMENTS:

FLEXIBILITY, RELAXATION MEDITATION:

ACTIVITY PERFORMED	MINUTES

ENERGY LEVEL:
☐ low
☐ medium
☐ high

NOTES/REMINDERS:

CALORIES BURNED:

TUESDAY

DATE:
/ /

WEIGHT:

WATER INTAKE:
# of 8oz. glasses
☐ ☐ ☐ ☐
☐ ☐ ☐ ☐

VITAMINS & SUPPLEMENTS:

_____
_____
_____
_____
_____
_____
_____
_____

ENERGY LEVEL:
☐ low
☐ medium
☐ high

CALORIES BURNED:

CARDIOVASCULAR EXERCISE:

EXERCISE TYPE	TIME/DISTANCE/PACE

STRENGTH TRAINING:

EXERCISE TYPE	WEIGHT	SETS	REPS

FLEXIBILITY, RELAXATION MEDITATION:

ACTIVITY PERFORMED	MINUTES

NOTES/REMINDERS:

DATE:
/ /

WEDNESDAY

CARDIOVASCULAR EXERCISE:

EXERCISE TYPE	TIME/DISTANCE/PACE
_____	_____
_____	_____
_____	_____

STRENGTH TRAINING:

EXERCISE TYPE	WEIGHT	SETS	REPS
_____			
_____			
_____			
_____			
_____			
_____			
_____			

FLEXIBILITY, RELAXATION MEDITATION:

ACTIVITY PERFORMED	MINUTES
_____	_____
_____	_____
_____	_____

NOTES/REMINDERS:

WEIGHT:

WATER INTAKE:
# of 8oz. glasses
☐ ☐ ☐ ☐
☐ ☐ ☐ ☐

VITAMINS & SUPPLEMENTS:

_____
_____
_____
_____
_____
_____
_____

ENERGY LEVEL:
☐ low
☐ medium
☐ high

CALORIES BURNED:

THURSDAY

DATE:
/ /

WEIGHT:

WATER INTAKE:
# of 8oz. glasses
☐ ☐ ☐ ☐
☐ ☐ ☐ ☐

VITAMINS & SUPPLEMENTS:

ENERGY LEVEL:
☐ low
☐ medium
☐ high

CALORIES BURNED:

CARDIOVASCULAR EXERCISE:

EXERCISE TYPE	TIME/DISTANCE/PACE

STRENGTH TRAINING:

EXERCISE TYPE	WEIGHT	SETS	REPS

FLEXIBILITY, RELAXATION MEDITATION:

ACTIVITY PERFORMED	MINUTES

NOTES/REMINDERS:

FRIDAY

CARDIOVASCULAR EXERCISE:

EXERCISE TYPE	TIME/DISTANCE/PACE

STRENGTH TRAINING:

EXERCISE TYPE	WEIGHT	SETS	REPS

FLEXIBILITY, RELAXATION MEDITATION:

ACTIVITY PERFORMED	MINUTES

NOTES/REMINDERS:

WEIGHT:

WATER INTAKE:
# of 8oz. glasses
☐ ☐ ☐ ☐
☐ ☐ ☐ ☐

VITAMINS & SUPPLEMENTS:

ENERGY LEVEL:
☐ low
☐ medium
☐ high

CALORIES BURNED:

SATURDAY

DATE: ___/___/___

WEIGHT:

WATER INTAKE:
# of 8oz. glasses
☐ ☐ ☐ ☐
☐ ☐ ☐ ☐

VITAMINS & SUPPLEMENTS:

_____

_____

_____

_____

_____

_____

_____

_____

ENERGY LEVEL:
☐ low
☐ medium
☐ high

CALORIES BURNED:

CARDIOVASCULAR EXERCISE:

EXERCISE TYPE	TIME/DISTANCE/PACE

STRENGTH TRAINING:

EXERCISE TYPE	WEIGHT	SETS	REPS

FLEXIBILITY, RELAXATION MEDITATION:

ACTIVITY PERFORMED	MINUTES

NOTES/REMINDERS:

DATE:

/ /

SUNDAY

CARDIOVASCULAR EXERCISE:

EXERCISE TYPE	TIME/DISTANCE/PACE

STRENGTH TRAINING:

EXERCISE TYPE	WEIGHT	SETS	REPS

FLEXIBILITY, RELAXATION MEDITATION:

ACTIVITY PERFORMED	MINUTES

NOTES/REMINDERS:

WEIGHT:

WATER INTAKE:
# of 8oz. glasses
☐ ☐ ☐ ☐
☐ ☐ ☐ ☐

VITAMINS & SUPPLEMENTS:

ENERGY LEVEL:
☐ low
☐ medium
☐ high

CALORIES BURNED:

End-of-the-Week WRAP-UP

WEEKLY ENERGY LEVEL:

☐ low ☐ med ☐ high

START WEIGHT:

END WEIGHT:

WEEKLY CALORIES BURNED:

DAYS I WORKED OUT:

☐ Mon. ☐ Tues. ☐ Wed. ☐ Thurs. ☐ Fri. ☐ Sat. ☐ Sun.

HOW I FELT THIS WEEK:

_____

_____

_____

_____

_____

GOALS FOR NEXT WEEK:

_____

_____

_____

_____

_____

NOTES/REMINDERS:

DATE:

MONDAY

_/_ /_

CARDIOVASCULAR EXERCISE:

EXERCISE TYPE	TIME/DISTANCE/PACE

STRENGTH TRAINING:

EXERCISE TYPE	WEIGHT	SETS	REPS

FLEXIBILITY, RELAXATION MEDITATION:

ACTIVITY PERFORMED	MINUTES

NOTES/REMINDERS:

WEIGHT:

WATER INTAKE:
# of 8oz. glasses
☐ ☐ ☐ ☐
☐ ☐ ☐ ☐

VITAMINS & SUPPLEMENTS:

ENERGY LEVEL:
☐ low
☐ medium
☐ high

CALORIES BURNED:

TUESDAY

DATE:
___/___/___

WEIGHT:

WATER INTAKE:
# of 8oz. glasses
☐ ☐ ☐ ☐
☐ ☐ ☐ ☐

**VITAMINS &
SUPPLEMENTS:**

_____

_____

_____

_____

_____

_____

ENERGY LEVEL:
☐ low
☐ medium
☐ high

**CALORIES
BURNED:**

CARDIOVASCULAR EXERCISE:

EXERCISE TYPE	TIME/DISTANCE/PACE

STRENGTH TRAINING:

EXERCISE TYPE	WEIGHT	SETS	REPS

FLEXIBILITY, RELAXATION MEDITATION:

ACTIVITY PERFORMED	MINUTES

NOTES/REMINDERS:

DATE: __/__/__

WEDNESDAY

CARDIOVASCULAR EXERCISE:

EXERCISE TYPE	TIME/DISTANCE/PACE

STRENGTH TRAINING:

EXERCISE TYPE	WEIGHT	SETS	REPS

FLEXIBILITY, RELAXATION MEDITATION:

ACTIVITY PERFORMED	MINUTES

NOTES/REMINDERS:

WEIGHT:

WATER INTAKE:
# of 8oz. glasses
☐ ☐ ☐ ☐
☐ ☐ ☐ ☐

VITAMINS & SUPPLEMENTS:

ENERGY LEVEL:
☐ low
☐ medium
☐ high

CALORIES BURNED:

THURSDAY

DATE: / /

WEIGHT:

WATER INTAKE:
# of 8oz. glasses
☐ ☐ ☐ ☐
☐ ☐ ☐ ☐

VITAMINS & SUPPLEMENTS:

_____

_____

_____

_____

_____

_____

_____

ENERGY LEVEL:
☐ low
☐ medium
☐ high

CALORIES BURNED:

CARDIOVASCULAR EXERCISE:

EXERCISE TYPE	TIME/DISTANCE/PACE

STRENGTH TRAINING:

EXERCISE TYPE	WEIGHT	SETS	REPS

FLEXIBILITY, RELAXATION MEDITATION:

ACTIVITY PERFORMED	MINUTES

NOTES/REMINDERS:

FRIDAY

CARDIOVASCULAR EXERCISE:

EXERCISE TYPE	TIME/DISTANCE/PACE

STRENGTH TRAINING:

EXERCISE TYPE	WEIGHT	SETS	REPS

FLEXIBILITY, RELAXATION MEDITATION:

ACTIVITY PERFORMED	MINUTES

NOTES/REMINDERS:

WEIGHT:

WATER INTAKE:
# of 8oz. glasses
☐ ☐ ☐ ☐
☐ ☐ ☐ ☐

**VITAMINS &
SUPPLEMENTS:**

ENERGY LEVEL:
☐ low
☐ medium
☐ high

**CALORIES
BURNED:**

SATURDAY

DATE: / /

WEIGHT:

WATER INTAKE:
# of 8oz. glasses
☐ ☐ ☐ ☐
☐ ☐ ☐ ☐

VITAMINS & SUPPLEMENTS:

_____
_____
_____
_____
_____
_____
_____

ENERGY LEVEL:
☐ low
☐ medium
☐ high

CALORIES BURNED:

CARDIOVASCULAR EXERCISE:

EXERCISE TYPE	TIME/DISTANCE/PACE

STRENGTH TRAINING:

EXERCISE TYPE	WEIGHT	SETS	REPS

FLEXIBILITY, RELAXATION MEDITATION:

ACTIVITY PERFORMED	MINUTES

NOTES/REMINDERS:

DATE: / /

SUNDAY

CARDIOVASCULAR EXERCISE:

EXERCISE TYPE	TIME/DISTANCE/PACE

STRENGTH TRAINING:

EXERCISE TYPE	WEIGHT	SETS	REPS

FLEXIBILITY, RELAXATION MEDITATION:

ACTIVITY PERFORMED	MINUTES

NOTES/REMINDERS:

WEIGHT:

WATER INTAKE:
# of 8oz. glasses
☐ ☐ ☐ ☐
☐ ☐ ☐ ☐

VITAMINS & SUPPLEMENTS:

ENERGY LEVEL:
☐ low
☐ medium
☐ high

CALORIES BURNED:

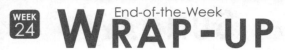

WEEKLY ENERGY LEVEL: **START WEIGHT:** **END WEIGHT:** **WEEKLY CALORIES BURNED:**

☐ low ☐ med ☐ high

DAYS I WORKED OUT:

☐ Mon. ☐ Tues. ☐ Wed. ☐ Thurs. ☐ Fri. ☐ Sat. ☐ Sun.

HOW I FELT THIS WEEK:

_____

_____

_____

_____

_____

GOALS FOR NEXT WEEK:

_____

_____

_____

_____

_____

NOTES/REMINDERS:

CARDIOVASCULAR EXERCISE:

EXERCISE TYPE	TIME/DISTANCE/PACE

STRENGTH TRAINING:

EXERCISE TYPE	WEIGHT	SETS	REPS

FLEXIBILITY, RELAXATION MEDITATION:

ACTIVITY PERFORMED	MINUTES

NOTES/REMINDERS:

WEIGHT:

WATER INTAKE:
# of 8oz. glasses
☐ ☐ ☐ ☐
☐ ☐ ☐ ☐

VITAMINS & SUPPLEMENTS:

ENERGY LEVEL:
☐ low
☐ medium
☐ high

CALORIES BURNED:

WEEK 25

TUESDAY

DATE: __/__/__

WEIGHT:

WATER INTAKE:
# of 8oz. glasses
☐ ☐ ☐ ☐
☐ ☐ ☐ ☐

**VITAMINS &
SUPPLEMENTS:**

_____

_____

_____

_____

_____

_____

_____

ENERGY LEVEL:
☐ low
☐ medium
☐ high

**CALORIES
BURNED:**

CARDIOVASCULAR EXERCISE:

EXERCISE TYPE	TIME/DISTANCE/PACE

STRENGTH TRAINING:

EXERCISE TYPE	WEIGHT	SETS	REPS

FLEXIBILITY, RELAXATION MEDITATION:

ACTIVITY PERFORMED	MINUTES

NOTES/REMINDERS:

WEDNESDAY

DATE: ___ / ___ / ___

CARDIOVASCULAR EXERCISE:

EXERCISE TYPE	TIME/DISTANCE/PACE

STRENGTH TRAINING:

EXERCISE TYPE	WEIGHT	SETS	REPS

FLEXIBILITY, RELAXATION MEDITATION:

ACTIVITY PERFORMED	MINUTES

NOTES/REMINDERS:

WEIGHT:

WATER INTAKE:
# of 8oz. glasses
☐ ☐ ☐ ☐
☐ ☐ ☐ ☐

VITAMINS & SUPPLEMENTS:

ENERGY LEVEL:
☐ low
☐ medium
☐ high

CALORIES BURNED:

THURSDAY

DATE: / /

WEIGHT:

WATER INTAKE:
# of 8oz. glasses
☐ ☐ ☐ ☐
☐ ☐ ☐ ☐

VITAMINS & SUPPLEMENTS:

_____

_____

_____

_____

_____

_____

_____

ENERGY LEVEL:
☐ low
☐ medium
☐ high

CALORIES BURNED:

CARDIOVASCULAR EXERCISE:

EXERCISE TYPE	TIME/DISTANCE/PACE

STRENGTH TRAINING:

EXERCISE TYPE	WEIGHT	SETS	REPS

FLEXIBILITY, RELAXATION MEDITATION:

ACTIVITY PERFORMED	MINUTES

NOTES/REMINDERS:

DATE:
/   /

FRIDAY

CARDIOVASCULAR EXERCISE:

EXERCISE TYPE	TIME/DISTANCE/PACE

STRENGTH TRAINING:

EXERCISE TYPE	WEIGHT	SETS	REPS

FLEXIBILITY, RELAXATION MEDITATION:

ACTIVITY PERFORMED	MINUTES

NOTES/REMINDERS:

WEIGHT:

WATER INTAKE:
# of 8oz. glasses
☐ ☐ ☐ ☐
☐ ☐ ☐ ☐

VITAMINS &
SUPPLEMENTS:

ENERGY LEVEL:
☐ low
☐ medium
☐ high

CALORIES
BURNED:

SATURDAY

DATE:
/ /

WEIGHT:

WATER INTAKE:
# of 8oz. glasses
☐ ☐ ☐ ☐
☐ ☐ ☐ ☐

**VITAMINS &
SUPPLEMENTS:**

ENERGY LEVEL:
☐ low
☐ medium
☐ high

**CALORIES
BURNED:**

CARDIOVASCULAR EXERCISE:

EXERCISE TYPE	TIME/DISTANCE/PACE

STRENGTH TRAINING:

EXERCISE TYPE	WEIGHT	SETS	REPS

FLEXIBILITY, RELAXATION MEDITATION:

ACTIVITY PERFORMED	MINUTES

NOTES/REMINDERS:

DATE:

  / /

SUNDAY

CARDIOVASCULAR EXERCISE:

EXERCISE TYPE	TIME/DISTANCE/PACE

STRENGTH TRAINING:

EXERCISE TYPE	WEIGHT	SETS	REPS

FLEXIBILITY, RELAXATION MEDITATION:

ACTIVITY PERFORMED	MINUTES

NOTES/REMINDERS:

WEIGHT:

WATER INTAKE:
# of 8oz. glasses
☐ ☐ ☐ ☐
☐ ☐ ☐ ☐

VITAMINS & SUPPLEMENTS:

ENERGY LEVEL:
☐ low
☐ medium
☐ high

CALORIES BURNED:

End-of-the-Week
WRAP-UP

WEEKLY ENERGY LEVEL:
☐ low ☐ med ☐ high

START WEIGHT:

END WEIGHT:

WEEKLY CALORIE: BURNED:

DAYS I WORKED OUT:
☐ Mon. ☐ Tues. ☐ Wed. ☐ Thurs. ☐ Fri. ☐ Sat. ☐ Sun.

HOW I FELT THIS WEEK:

_____

_____

_____

_____

_____

GOALS FOR NEXT WEEK:

_____

_____

_____

_____

_____

NOTES/REMINDERS:

DATE:

/ /

MONDAY

WEEK 26

CARDIOVASCULAR EXERCISE:

EXERCISE TYPE	TIME/DISTANCE/PACE

STRENGTH TRAINING:

EXERCISE TYPE	WEIGHT	SETS	REPS

FLEXIBILITY, RELAXATION MEDITATION:

ACTIVITY PERFORMED	MINUTES

NOTES/REMINDERS:

WEIGHT:

WATER INTAKE:
# of 8oz. glasses
☐ ☐ ☐ ☐
☐ ☐ ☐ ☐

VITAMINS & SUPPLEMENTS:

ENERGY LEVEL:
☐ low
☐ medium
☐ high

CALORIES BURNED:

TUESDAY

DATE: / /

WEIGHT:

WATER INTAKE:
# of 8oz. glasses

☐ ☐ ☐ ☐
☐ ☐ ☐ ☐

VITAMINS & SUPPLEMENTS:

_____
_____
_____
_____
_____
_____
_____

ENERGY LEVEL:
☐ low
☐ medium
☐ high

CALORIES BURNED:

CARDIOVASCULAR EXERCISE:

EXERCISE TYPE	TIME/DISTANCE/PACE

STRENGTH TRAINING:

EXERCISE TYPE	WEIGHT	SETS	REPS

FLEXIBILITY, RELAXATION MEDITATION:

ACTIVITY PERFORMED	MINUTES

NOTES/REMINDERS:

DATE: / /

WEDNESDAY

CARDIOVASCULAR EXERCISE:

EXERCISE TYPE	TIME/DISTANCE/PACE

STRENGTH TRAINING:

EXERCISE TYPE	WEIGHT	SETS	REPS

FLEXIBILITY, RELAXATION MEDITATION:

ACTIVITY PERFORMED	MINUTES

NOTES/REMINDERS:

WEIGHT:

WATER INTAKE:
# of 8oz. glasses
☐ ☐ ☐ ☐
☐ ☐ ☐ ☐

**VITAMINS &
SUPPLEMENTS:**

ENERGY LEVEL:
☐ low
☐ medium
☐ high

**CALORIES
BURNED:**

THURSDAY

DATE: / /

WEIGHT:

WATER INTAKE:
# of 8oz. glasses
☐ ☐ ☐ ☐
☐ ☐ ☐ ☐

VITAMINS & SUPPLEMENTS:

_____
_____
_____
_____
_____
_____
_____
_____

ENERGY LEVEL:
☐ low
☐ medium
☐ high

CALORIES BURNED:

CARDIOVASCULAR EXERCISE:

EXERCISE TYPE	TIME/DISTANCE/PACE

STRENGTH TRAINING:

EXERCISE TYPE	WEIGHT	SETS	REPS

FLEXIBILITY, RELAXATION MEDITATION:

ACTIVITY PERFORMED	MINUTES

NOTES/REMINDERS:

FRIDAY

CARDIOVASCULAR EXERCISE:

EXERCISE TYPE	TIME/DISTANCE/PACE

STRENGTH TRAINING:

EXERCISE TYPE	WEIGHT	SETS	REPS

FLEXIBILITY, RELAXATION MEDITATION:

ACTIVITY PERFORMED	MINUTES

NOTES/REMINDERS:

WEIGHT:

WATER INTAKE:
# of 8oz. glasses
☐ ☐ ☐ ☐
☐ ☐ ☐ ☐

**VITAMINS &
SUPPLEMENTS:**

ENERGY LEVEL:
☐ low
☐ medium
☐ high

**CALORIES
BURNED:**

SATURDAY

DATE:
__ / __ / __

WEIGHT:

WATER INTAKE:
# of 8oz. glasses
☐ ☐ ☐ ☐
☐ ☐ ☐ ☐

VITAMINS & SUPPLEMENTS:

_____
_____
_____
_____
_____
_____
_____

ENERGY LEVEL:
☐ low
☐ medium
☐ high

CALORIES BURNED:

CARDIOVASCULAR EXERCISE:

EXERCISE TYPE	TIME/DISTANCE/PACE

STRENGTH TRAINING:

EXERCISE TYPE	WEIGHT	SETS	REPS

FLEXIBILITY, RELAXATION MEDITATION:

ACTIVITY PERFORMED	MINUTES

NOTES/REMINDERS:

CARDIOVASCULAR EXERCISE:

EXERCISE TYPE   **TIME/DISTANCE/PACE**

_____ _____

_____ _____

_____ _____

STRENGTH TRAINING:

EXERCISE TYPE **WEIGHT** **SETS** **REPS**

FLEXIBILITY, RELAXATION MEDITATION:

ACTIVITY PERFORMED **MINUTES**

_____ _____

_____ _____

_____ _____

NOTES/REMINDERS:

WEIGHT:

WATER INTAKE:
# of 8oz. glasses
☐ ☐ ☐ ☐
☐ ☐ ☐ ☐

**VITAMINS &
SUPPLEMENTS:**

_____

_____

_____

_____

_____

_____

_____

_____

ENERGY LEVEL:
☐ low
☐ medium
☐ high

**CALORIES
BURNED:**

End-of-the-Week WRAP-UP

WEEKLY ENERGY LEVEL:	START WEIGHT:	END WEIGHT:	WEEKLY CALORIES BURNED:
☐ low ☐ med ☐ high			

DAYS I WORKED OUT:

☐ Mon. ☐ Tues. ☐ Wed. ☐ Thurs. ☐ Fri. ☐ Sat. ☐ Sun.

HOW I FELT THIS WEEK:

_____

_____

_____

_____

GOALS FOR NEXT WEEK:

_____

_____

_____

_____

_____

NOTES/REMINDERS: